DANCE ADVENTURES

True Stories About Dancing Abroad

Senior Editor: Megan Taylor Morrison
Assistant Editor: Elisa Koshkina

Follow us on Instagram:

@dancetravelabroad
@megantaylormorrison

Join our Facebook group:

Dance Travelers: Explore the World Through Movement

ISBN 978-1-7354842-4-2 (hardcover)
ISBN 978-1-7354842-5-9 (softcover)

Printed in the United States of America

DEDICATIONS

To my dear friend and mentor, Sarah Lee,
Your dedication to your art, vivacious spirit, huge heart, fortitude, and awesome hairstyles inspire me to live more boldly. Your life is one great dance adventure, and you embody what it means to have a lifelong commitment to a calling. I cannot thank you enough for coordinating the grandest dance adventure of my life. It forever changed me. I can't wait to see you in Guinea someday soon.

To my fellow dance adventurers,
Someday, we will sit around a bonfire and tell stories all night long.

PRAISE FOR
DANCE ADVENTURES

"*Armchair travel has never had it so good! Dropping into these cultural adventures is like landing feet first on the most dynamic dance floors around the globe. Each carefully curated story gives a dancer's-eye view of the people, places, and practices that enrich our planet.*"

—Mark Metz, publisher of Conscious Dancer Magazine and founder of The Dance First Association

"*Fun and engaging, Dance Adventures takes you on a playful journey around the world led by dancers who use their art form to deepen their connections to other cultures and to themselves.*"

—Kelly Lewis, founder of Women's Travel Fest

"*This book is indispensable in light of the current social momentum with regard to Black lives and the dismantling of violent systems. Many of the stories portray the experiences of individuals in whom multiple languages, customs, and spaces coexist, and for whom dance is the unifying factor.*"

—Moncell Durden, Assistant Professor of Practice, USC Kaufman School of Dance

"*A heartwarming, humorous, and enlightening anthology, Dance Adventures is a pivotal text capturing rich narratives that can help students prepare for the unknown and integrate their own life-changing experiences from dancing abroad.*"

—Rick Southerland, MFA, Associate Professor of Dance, Goucher College, past president of the National Dance Education Organization (2016-2018)

"*Dance Adventures* contains beautiful moments of transformation and connection through dance—a wonderful extension of Meg's own mission. The anthology's writers create a strong case for using dance to understand the world."

—Mickela Mallozzi, Emmy® Award-winning TV host of *Bare Feet with Mickela Mallozzi*

"*I was captivated by Megan Taylor Morrison's Dance Adventures! This vibrant and emotionally explorative collection of tales captures the power of dance in a way that transcends the stage.*"

—Aisha Mitchell, Alvin Ailey American Dance Theater member (2008–2013), Broadway soloist in *Oklahoma* (2019), and featured performer in *The Lion King* (2013–2018)

"*In a pandemic-gripped world full of restrictions and uncertainties, Dance Adventures offers readers an escape. This diverse collection of stories encourages us to dream of embodied explorations, and once more to discover human connectivity through dance and movement.*"

—Jen Peters, dance writer, performer, and teacher

"*A must-read for anyone who is ready for an incredible adventure! Enjoy stories of family, community, culture, love, teaching, and learning with a unique, global perspective.*"

—Dr. Karen Campbell Kuebler, dance educator, dance historian, and adjunct faculty, Towson University

"*Touching and emotionally satisfying, these stories woke up a part of me that had almost become dormant due t0 current events. It made me remember how dancing makes me feel: hypnotized in the trance of time, in dreamland until the music stops...*"

—Daniel Erijo, accountant, dance influencer, and founder of Dancing in the Air✈ (Facebook group)

TABLE OF CONTENTS

FOREWORD
Tanja "La Alemana" Kensinger

"The journey of a thousand miles begins with a single step," is a quote generally attributed to the ancient Chinese philosopher Lao Tzu. For us to begin the adventure we seek, we must take the first, single step. Yours may be reading this book.

I took the first steps in my own dance adventure at the age of three in Wuerzburg, Germany. My mother was a ballroom dancer there before and during her pregnancy, so I basically danced out of her womb.

From the time I was a child, whenever I heard music, my body moved on its own. Whether it was music on the radio at home or from street musicians during a walk downtown, I always danced. And I danced hard. As I moved into adolescence, dance became a way to express myself before I knew how to put words to my emotions.

I believe many people have a similar experience. No matter your age or background, music and dance have the power to get deep inside your soul, and they can inspire you to express yourself when words seem to fail. Not many things on Earth have power like that.

Music and dance can also bring together people from all walks of life. I've witnessed this firsthand. Although I don't speak Spanish, I have had the incredible opportunity to be part of the Latin dance community as a professional dancer since 2005. Dance has allowed me to communicate with people around the world without having to utter one single syllable.

One memory I cherish is from an event in Salerno, Italy, at which I was hired to teach, perform, and social dance with the attendees. Throughout the night, Jorge and I were social dancing and switching partners about every 45 seconds.

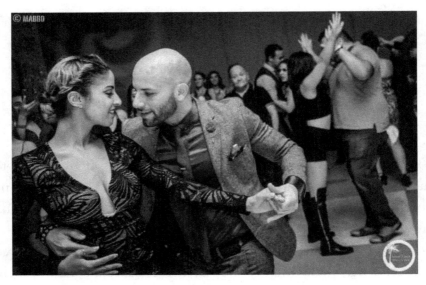

Tanja dances bachata with her husband and
dance partner, Jorge "Ataca" Burgos
Photo credit: Michael "Mabbo" Mabborang

This continued until I started dancing with one young gentleman. He was feeling the music, but also tapping his fingers on my back. I thought this was odd, but I didn't pay it too much mind... until I saw that he was wearing a cochlear implant. He was deaf!

At that very moment, I thought, *Wow! This is incredible. He can maybe only hear certain sounds, but he is able to keep a beat much better than some hearing dancers I've known.*

Needless to say, I didn't want to switch partners after 45 seconds. We continued our dance until the song ended. Before we went our separate ways, we signed, "Thank you," to each other. I was left feeling touched and inspired. This is just one example of how I've been able to experience people and cultures in beautiful and mind-opening ways through dance.

When I first read some of the stories from *Dance Adventures*, I was almost brought to tears. The book demonstrates what I have believed for so long: there are no limits to what music and dance can provide us. Meg has carefully and thoughtfully selected stories that reflect the power of dance to shape the way a person experiences life. Her mission to share tales of individuals' dance travels around the world is something to be truly admired.

In this, the first book of its kind whose subject is solely dance adventures, each story will touch your heart in a different way. You will read about dancers finding themselves through music and movement. You'll find out how dance helped several authors shed self-doubt and allow themselves to be vulnerable. You'll discover that dance is a universal language, stronger than any cultural divide. You'll learn that the world is not such a scary place, but instead is full of beauty, peace, and unity.

I hope not only that you enjoy these stories as much as I have, but that they open you to a part of yourself that may have been locked away, or that you never knew existed. May this book inspire you to take the next step toward an adventure of your own, whether it's dancing in a faraway location or finding the courage to pursue your goals.

Dance is powerful. If we listen to the music, let go, and allow ourselves to dance together toward new horizons, life can be a truly magnificent experience.

Just dance!
Tanja "La Alemana" Kensinger
Acclaimed bachata dancer and instructor

About the author: Tanja Kensinger, also known as "La Alemana" in the international Latin dance scene, became a professional dancer in 2005. It wasn't until 2008, however, that her career took off. That year, she met Jorge "Ataca" Burgos, now her husband and dance partner. Tanja and Jorge longed to be professional salsa dancers, but they were both beginners with salsa choreography. Knowing they needed to showcase their partnership, the duo decided to put together a bachata routine, since it was a style they danced well together. Their breakout bachata performance has become the most viewed choreographed YouTube bachata dance video of all time, with more than 99 million views. La Alemana and Ataca have since become the most recognizable bachata dance couple around the world.

INTRODUCTION

Megan Taylor Morrison

Dear Readers,

Our world is a much different place than it was when this project began. This year, 2020, is a time of dissidence, when we are simultaneously experiencing a great pause and great change. As COVID-19 requires us to spend far more time at home, we are also beginning a new, powerful chapter on achieving racial equality in the United States.

Like many people around the world, I have been inspired by current events to think more deeply about my beliefs, as well as my endeavors. With everything going on, I had to ask myself: why publish a book about dance travel now?

I came up with two answers.

The first: I believe adventures that fill us with wonder are critical to our wellbeing. Yet, for many of us right now, life-giving experiences are in short supply. The things we love – such as attending incredible dance performances, going to dance classes, or hugging people within our dance communities – feel far away.

The second: After the death of George Floyd, I realized this book needed to be part of how I participate in the change I want to see in the US. To make sure our stories represented cultures in a respectful way and did not perpetuate harmful stereotypes, I hired a perspective consultant to review our authors' work. By choosing contributors from many different walks of life, I am taking a stand for more diversity in the predominantly white-washed travel writing industry.

As stories from these authors came in, I began to recognize themes in their writing. Thus, this book is divided into four parts:

1. Roots: Join Makeda Kumasi, Ted Samuel, Courtney Celeste Spears, and Kara Nepomuceno as they travel to a country connected to their heritage.
2. Finding Community: No friends? No problem! Connecting with others through a shared love of movement helped Damilare Adeyeri, Carolyn McPherson, Tina Shield, Gabrielle Brigida Macalintal, and Melaina Spitzer find their place.
3. Unexpected Experiences: In these stories, Alex Milweski, Nneya Richardson, Laurie Bonner Baker, Peter Benjamin, and Natalie Preddie are surprised and enriched by what they discover through their dance travels.
4. Personal Development: Lisa Josefsson, Khalila Fordham, Zsuzsi Kapas, Helen Styring Tocci, and I share stories about how dancing abroad challenged us to live with more self-expression, grow our self-love, heal old traumas, or otherwise evolve in positive ways.

It has been my absolute privilege to work with each contributor to craft an engaging story that honors the power of dance travel. I commend all of the authors for their creativity, dedication, and commitment to this anthology.

On behalf of everyone involved with this project, thank you for your support. We sincerely hope you are touched and inspired by the stories we share.

Embrace the Adventure,

Meg
Senior Editor of Dance Adventures

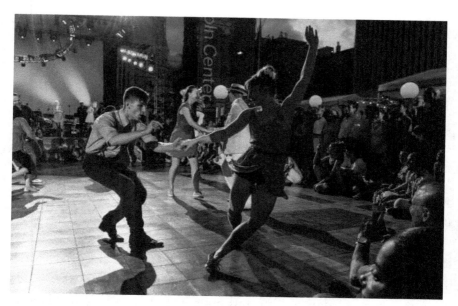

Rafal Pustelny (left) and Megan Taylor Morrison (right)
dance lindy hop at Lincoln Center in New York City
Photo credit: Nanette Melville

OUR COMMITMENTS

Celebrate the power of dance: Each story highlights a way that dance can uplift the human spirit, invite us to challenge our assumptions, and ultimately transform us into better versions of ourselves. Through this book, we celebrate how dance can give us access to wisdom, community, and unbridled delight, no matter where we are on the planet.

Prioritize diversity and inclusion: The fact that we can offer stories from many different viewpoints is a further testament to the far-reaching power of dance. Our authors come from different religious, ethnic, and socioeconomic backgrounds, and our stories take place all over the world. There are also – of course! – many different dance forms represented in the following pages. *Dance Adventures* celebrates dance traditions across North and South America, Africa, Europe, and Asia. We welcome stories from everyone and from every corner of the Earth, while recognizing the limitations on the stories we tell as an English-based project. If you are interested in having your work published in our next anthology, you'll find information at the end of this book about how to submit your story.

Encourage awareness and positive change in the travel industry: We acknowledge there is inherent privilege in being able to travel, that the tourist experience isn't the same for everyone, and that most travel publications have far too few BIPOC contributors. We are committed to including a wide range of voices in this anthology so that readers can experience travel through many different lenses.

Learn from the wisdom of others: Humility is a theme in our stories. Some authors arrive at their destination ready to learn as much as possible from new mentors or the region they're visiting. Others arrive with their ego or fear leading the way. You'll watch how their experience evolves. Authors learn that their fears were misplaced, or that they had more to learn than they could have guessed. We want this book to demonstrate the ways in which we can all learn from one another and the goodness that pervades the world.

Seek feedback: We are grateful to our perspective consultant, Dr. LaToya T. Brackett, as well as to the authors who had their stories read by their mentors. We're also appreciative of our proofreaders and those who gave feedback about the stories and book design. This helped us in our goal of sharing about dancers, culture bearers, and dance traditions with nuance and care. And, while we've done our best with this first edition, we know we're not perfect. There's always room for improvement and lessons to learn. If you believe there is something we could do better, please send your recommendations to megan@megantaylormorrison.com.

Invite further education: Dances and traditions are dynamic, and we invite you to learn more about any topic that inspires you through your own research and travel, as well as through the resources the authors have included at the end of each story.

PART 1: ROOTS

"If you don't know your history, then you don't know anything.
You are a leaf that doesn't know it is part of a tree."
-Michael Crichton

There are many meaningful ways to explore and build a connection to your cultural heritage. You might study a language, learn to cook traditional dishes, or read about cultural practices in the birthplace of your ancestors.

For many dancers, however, movement is the most powerful avenue for understanding, celebrating, or sharing their roots. In this, the opening section of our book, authors recount stories about dance adventures in locations tied to their family history.

While some authors are visiting a country for the first time, others consider their destination a second home. Through their experiences, these writers explore their connection to their past, their identity in the present, and their desires for the future.

Performing My Culture

The Journey of an Indian-American Folk Dancer
A. Ted Samuel, Ph.D.

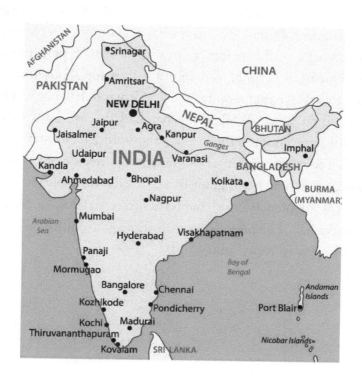

About the author: Since 2003, Ted has studied South Indian classical and folk dances, integrating a mastery of technique with broader anthropological investigations of performers' lives. During this time, Ted found a love for *Karagattam*, a Tamil folk dance that requires the performer to balance a brass pot on their head. To date, he has had the opportunity to perform Karagattam in the United States, India, Pakistan, and Nepal. Ted currently serves as the deputy director of Oberlin Shansi, an exchange program based at Oberlin College. This story was adapted from a chapter written for *Shaping Minds: Multicultural Literature,* an anthology published by Authorspress in New Delhi.

I landed at the Chennai International Airport on a muggy night in August, 2003. Jet lag and dehydration left me in a complete stupor as I waited in the long, disorganized immigration and customs lines. Even though it was nearly midnight, I was overwhelmed by the heat and bustling confusion. I was in over my head, and I did not belong.

No more than thirty seconds after I claimed my luggage, a stocky, middle-aged porter with a classically manicured South Indian mustache approached me, speaking in rapid Tamil. Despite my dazed expression and my North American clothing (complete with oversized hiking boots and a Mardi Gras-themed t-shirt from New Orleans), he saw my black hair, brown skin, and typical Tamil facial features and assumed I was a local.

This was my chance to prove myself. For several months prior to my arrival, I had been studying Tamil intensively and had become proficient enough to converse with my parents and grandparents in my family's mother tongue. But this particular porter was speaking too rapidly for me to understand. I immediately responded, using the best Tamil accent I could muster, "*Enakku Tamil Pidikaathu.*"

The porter gave me a confused look and immediately switched to English.

"Please, sir," he said. "I can take the bag."

I uttered a succinct, "No thanks," and headed toward the baggage claim exit. As I walked away, I replayed this interaction in my head repeatedly. How had he known I was American? It wasn't until I walked through the exit doors that I realized my revealing mistake. I meant to say, "I do not understand Tamil," or, "*Enakku Tamil Puriyaathu,*" but ended up telling the porter that I do not *like* Tamil.

At that moment, my aspirations of seamless integration into "the motherland" were shattered. Needless to say, I was embarrassed. I wondered how I could have messed up so quickly. I also questioned why I had deemed it necessary to communicate the fact that I did not know the Tamil language well while speaking... Tamil. Had I just spoken to the porter in English, I could have avoided this snafu.

Even though it was only the porter who had experienced this

moment with me, I felt as if an entire audience had witnessed my mistake. As I replayed the scene in my mind, I imagined the lights around me had dimmed, and I was an actor on stage who had forgotten all his lines. The audience sat silently, waiting for my next move. As the awkward moment dragged on, I imagined snickers and giggles coming from the imaginary spectators. I felt like I had failed miserably in proving my "Tamilness."

Claiming my heritage had never posed much of a problem prior to this experience, because I had rarely ever been tested. Having grown up in a rural village in the Appalachian foothills, I'd never had to prove that I was Indian, much less South Indian. Granted, some of my peers had assumed I was Black, Mexican, or even Chinese, but when I had explained that my parents had come from a country called India, they had usually accepted it as the truth.

No one had ever tested me by asking about Indian politics or contemporary cinema. Had they done so, they would have discovered that my knowledge of Indian history was limited to anecdotes about well-known historical figures like Emperor Shah Jahan and Mahatma Gandhi, which I had found in my sixth-grade social studies textbook. I could barely recognize Tamil movie stars like MGR or Rajinikanth, and would not have been able to discuss the famed political career of the former. I had no idea how much I didn't know. I could not speak to India's linguistic, cultural, and religious diversity. Tamil Nadu, in particular, was little more than an imaginary place where everyone looked like me, no one made fun of my parents' accents, and – on particularly special occasions – an elephant would saunter throughout the alleys of my neighborhood.

Now here I was in South India, about to realize how much more I could learn. Part of my decision to study abroad here was a desire to reconnect with my roots. However, I affirmed this path because of my growing academic, professional, and artistic interest in the region. In college, I had taken several classes on South Asian history, literature, and film, and I knew that actually studying in India would be the next step in my academic career. I had enrolled in the University of

Wisconsin's College Year in India program knowing that I would have the chance to conduct my own research, intensively study Tamil, and – perhaps most importantly – immerse myself in a culture that seemed both inborn and foreign to me.

I wish I could say that my initial encounter at the airport was my only slipup, but that would be a massive understatement. Two months into the program, I fell out of a slowly moving bus and tumbled to the side of the street where a very real, live audience watched with both concern and amusement. By the time the first semester ended, I had called my landlord no fewer than seven times to help me into my apartment, because I continued to lock myself out. And in yet another linguistic faux pas, I confused the Tamil words for mosquito and fart – *kosu* and *kusu*, respectively – when talking to a group of neighborhood children. These episodes of incompetence were interspersed with bouts of fevers, food poisoning, and one nasty case of dysentery.

Even so, my initial time in India was extremely rewarding in academic, professional, and personal arenas. My Tamil improved drastically; I had embarked upon research on Tamil Nadu's transgender population, and I even managed to sport a classic South Indian mustache for several months. As time progressed, people mistook me for a local more often. As my confidence grew, I started playing the part of a Tamil student and scholar with greater ease and panache.

But the self-doubt never fully dissipated. I still viewed my endeavors as those of an American trying to assimilate into a culture where he did not completely fit in. No matter what I looked like, how good my Tamil was, or how many local friends I made, I was still a foreigner in a region that my parents had once called home. I still brushed my teeth and rinsed my mouth with bottled water. Crossing roads still caused occasional pangs of panic. Sometimes, I chose to wear my Mardi Gras t-shirt and oversized hiking boots because they made me feel comfortable.

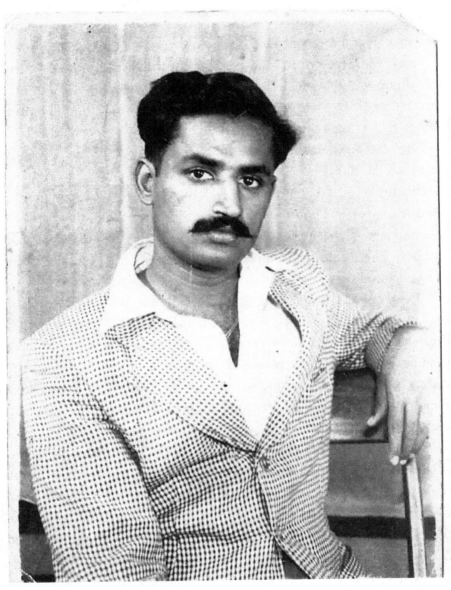

A photo of the author's grandfather, Bernard Chinnappa, with a
Tamil mustache
Photo credit: Anonymous

There was one aspect of my studies, however, that allowed me to veer away from my Americanness in favor of more local, Tamil sensibilities: becoming involved in the performing arts. As part of the University of Wisconsin's program's curriculum, students could opt to take tutorials in handicraft production, yoga, music, or dance. Having been an avid comedic performer in high school plays and variety shows, I knew I wanted to study a South Indian performance art form that would let me capitalize on my buffoonish stage presence, allow me to explore local cultural dynamics of artisan communities, and broaden my skills as an entertainer.

The answer was Karagattam, a Tamil folk art in which the performer is required to balance a decorated brass pot on their head while dancing and sometimes executing circus-like stunts that could incorporate fire, ladders, and literal pins and needles. Karagattam has a long history in Tamil Nadu, and has evolved significantly over the centuries. Religious iterations of the art form, known as *Sakthi Karagattam*, were historically reserved for ceremonial offerings to the goddess Mariamman. However, in the early 20th century, a secular version of the dance, *Attak Karagattam*, emerged with the popularization of Tamil film and other regional folk arts. Whereas highly manicured classical Indian dances like Bharata Natyam gained national and international recognition, Karagattam maintained its popularity among local, agrarian communities. The dance was not relegated to formal stages or the inner sanctums of temples; it could be performed in public in open-air venues like village squares and marketplaces.

My inspiration for learning the art form had come from the hit Tamil movie *Karagattakaran*, a romantic comedy that depicted the courtship between two Karagattam performers from neighboring villages. I had watched the 1989 blockbuster in a Tamil class in Madison the summer prior to the UW program. Though I had only understood about fifty percent of the plot, the musical numbers had drawn me in. The punchy drumbeats and the fast-paced melodies laid the backdrop for energetic choreography in which the dancers integrated complex footwork, droll facial expressions, and precise, uninterrupted balance.

17

Karagattam, as depicted in this movie, left little room for subtlety. It was fun. It was entertaining. It was quirky.

The movie planted a seed, and I began to explore the possibility of enrolling in a Karagattam tutorial during the UW program. Through online research and conversations with the program's staff after I arrived in India, I learned that the dance allowed space for improvisation. As I had been less than perfect at learning choreography during my heyday in high school musicals, I was intrigued by the freedom that Karagattam could afford. I also found out that some dancers incorporated humor and playful lewdness, as evidenced by routines that featured not-so-coy acts of chopping phallic fruits and vegetables like bananas, carrots, and cucumbers. Karagattam appealed to my comedic instincts in a way that few other dance styles would. Furthermore, given its relatively low profile outside of South India, this study abroad program offered the opportunity to learn an art form that most Americans would not even have the chance to watch.

I also had hesitations. In particular, I questioned my ability to balance a heavy object on my head. Either the brass pot would stay on my head or it wouldn't. In this situation, I would not be able to ad-lib or smile through a mistake. There was also the distinct possibility that my skull was too pointy, or that I was too inherently clumsy to be successful. If I studied Karagattam, I might be giving up the opportunity to learn something that didn't require an audience, like sari-weaving or traditional pottery. But no matter how much I tried to talk myself out of taking the tutorial, I couldn't shake the desire to push my comfort zone as an entertainer.

The University of Wisconsin program's staff provided me with the best teacher possible. Madurai Veeran was an accomplished performer of several different styles of Tamil folk performance and South Indian martial arts. By the time I began working with him, he had a resume that spanned India, and had mentored dozens of local and international students. He also came from a long line of iconic artists. His father, Om Periyaswami – arguably the most famed Karagattam dancer of his generation – performed all over India, Europe, and even the United

States.

My first Karagattam lesson was only a minor disaster. Rather than focusing on dance steps, my teacher wanted me to work on balance. He filled a sturdy paper cone with sand, sealed the open end, placed it on my head, and told me to walk around. He had me walk in circles, figure eights, and up and down stairs. That poor paper cone took a beating that day, falling off my head at least two dozen times. By the time the lesson was over, its edges were worn, and its shape completely mutilated.

Every time I felt that cone slip off my head, my nerves crackled in frustration. I began to worry that Madurai Veeran would get annoyed at my clumsiness and general ineptitude. But he was remarkably patient and supportive. Even though we faced communication gaps because he was not fluent in English and my Tamil was still improving, I understood my teacher's primary message during that first lesson: performing this dance would be more about my state of mind than about perfect technique. He wanted me to stop being so hard on myself every time that sand-filled paper cone wobbled. He told me to relax and simply believe that I could do it. His advice was much easier said than done, but it was exactly what I needed to hear.

As I continued with Karagattam, my balance improved drastically. I graduated from a paper cone to a brass pot within a few lessons. Though I was excited about my progress, I quickly realized the dangers of balancing a heavy brass pot on one's head while trying to maneuver around a stage with even a shred of grace. On more than one occasion, my toes felt the crushing defeat of my inability to keep that pot from falling to the ground. But, with the encouragement of my teacher, I overcame the minor injuries and learned the dance steps.

Within three months, I knew three dance routines and was primed to tackle my first stunt: a feat of balance that would make audiences gasp and then (if I did it properly) laugh with delight. The stunt was part of a playful but difficult routine called the Sari-Tying Act.

Within this performance, a male solo dancer coyly flirts with the audience while dancing next to a six-yard sari laid out full-length on the ground. Next, with the utmost precision and care, the performer lies on top of the sari while keeping his neck and torso elevated to prevent the pot from falling off his head. Slowly, he tucks a corner of the sari into his belt and carefully rolls over while keeping his head upright. After making a complete 360-degree turn, the dancer folds the sari into pleats with his right hand and continues to tuck the remaining fabric into his belt. After one more roll, he drapes the remaining fabric over his shoulder and stands up wearing a perfectly tied sari. The sheer difficulty of this act is only enhanced by the comedic drag performance that follows. Saris are, after all, traditionally worn by women.

When I first saw Madurai Veeran demonstrate this act in one of our lessons, my jaw literally dropped. He made it look so easy, as if the pot was an extension of his head and he dressed himself everyday while skillfully rolling on the ground. My amazement led to bemused confusion. Did he honestly expect me to perform the same stunt in spite of my limited experience? He was almost comically adamant that I would do this stunt for my first performance, which was less than a month away. Furthermore, he insisted that I would do it well. As much as I appreciated his confidence, I thought he was insane.

My first attempt was a flop, as were my second and third. It took several tries before I could make it through half of the routine without the pot tumbling to the ground. But, as I continued to practice, I became more confident. Rather than expending my energy by stressing out about how I might fail, I started listening to Madurai Veeran's advice. I acted as if I knew exactly what I was doing. I believed that I would be able to perform the stunt and do it well. My dancing improved.

Of course, believing in yourself while practicing is one thing. Performing in front of a live audience is another. In spite of my newfound confidence, I felt butterflies the size of bats in my stomach before my debut. I wondered what the audience expected of me. Would they smirk at the audacity of an American doing a centuries-old dance after only studying it for four months? Did they imagine that I'd fail? All of the feelings of self-doubt and anxiety that I had felt in the Chennai airport during my first day in India rushed back. I was risking yet another humiliation, but this time there really *was* an audience who would judge me.

As I stood in front of the crowd and the music played, instinct and confidence took over. The entire performance felt surreal. Perhaps it was a result of the skill I'd developed or my hyper-focus from the adrenaline, but the pot rested comfortably on my head as if it were a genuine extension of my body. There were moments when my footwork was a bit sloppy and times when I could have played up the comedy better. But judging from the claps, hoots, gasps, and laughter from the audience, I had made my newfound community in India proud. As for me, I felt like I had proven myself. I had succeeded in something truly Tamil, and I felt like I belonged.

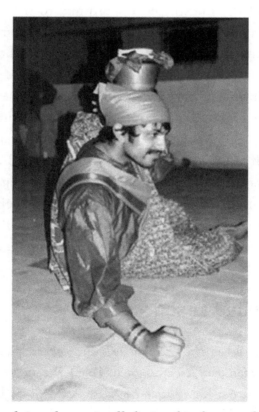

The author doing the sari roll during his first performance in
Madurai, India
Photo credit: Anonymous

After this first recital, I knew I had to keep performing and improving my craft. While in India, I gave demonstrations and performed at NGOs, orphanages, and even small family gatherings. When I returned to the United States for my final year of college, I continued to choreograph new numbers and showcase my dance at multicultural functions. After winning a Fulbright Fellowship in 2005 to continue my research on the Tamil transgender community, I still found time to dance at various events. I was even invited to perform at the 2006 Fulbright Alumni Conference in Islamabad, and at the International Theatre Institute in Kathmandu.

Within a few short years, I had gone from a curious American who was interested in Tamil folk arts to a genuine international performer. Moreover, I had the unexpected opportunity to serve as an artistic ambassador for a piece of Tamil culture. Not bad for someone who had mistakenly claimed that he did not like Tamil at the Chennai airport!

Years after my first independent journey to India, I still take the words of my Karagattam teacher, Madurai Veeran, to heart. Whether I am interacting with Tamil family members or challenging myself to try something new, I do not dwell on my mistakes or faux pas. I have realized that self-belief goes a long way. To this day, I am faced with embarrassing moments like the one I experienced at the Chennai airport in August of 2003. I still know that feeling of being an actor on stage who has forgotten his lines and (cultural) cues. But rather than allowing embarrassment to overwhelm me, I persevere. My show must go on.

Recommended resources:

Editor's note: When I reached out to Ted about additional resources, he shared that most additional resources are in Tamil. We are grateful to have his story so that more about Karagattam can be shared with English speakers. He also recommends the following YouTube videos:

ATKT.in (Director). (2019, September 7). *Karakattam Folk Dance*

Showcase by Sathaye College Students | Malhar 2019 [Video file]. Retrieved July 7, 2020, from https://www.youtube.com/watch?v=ne4LBs52QD4

Bright, S. (Director). (2018, November 6). *Karagattam..The Tamil folk dance....my first stage in kalai kaviri...* [Video file]. Retrieved July 7, 2020, from https://www.youtube.com/watch?v=i5QLOVpYmjwgabrielle

SunTV Network (Director). (2012, January 11). *Karakattam by Kalaimamani Thenmozhi in Vayalodu Vilaiyadi* [Video file]. Retrieved July 7, 2020, from https://www.youtube.com/watch?v=Lx1_eIWG4EI

WE RETURN

Makeda Kumasi

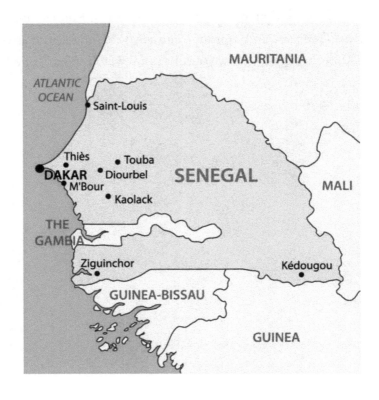

About the author: Makeda Kumasi is a multi-talented artist and teacher who has received numerous awards and recognitions. She was a California Arts Scholar, and has also been honored with the Ida Mae Holland Playwright's Award, the Top Spoken Word Artists Award at the Black Business Expo in Los Angeles, and the Phyllis E. Williams' Artist Grant.

Makeda is the founder of WE 3 PRODUCTIONS, and teaches fine arts through The Sesh Project, a program designed to teach youth the art of the Jali, who are African oral historians and artisans. Makeda is a playwright and the author of two books, as well as the producer of a documentary short.

Makeda has danced for two prominent Southern California-based African dance ensembles, and performed in musicals including *Bye Bye Birdie* and *Grease*.

She has been featured on MTV's *Starting Over*, BET's *Fly Poet*, the first season of *So You Think You Can Dance?*, and has appeared in independent films and community theater productions. Currently, Makeda teaches for the Department of Dance and the Department of Theater, Film, and Digital Production at the University of California, Riverside. Makeda received an MFA in theater from the University of Southern California and a master's in education from the University of Phoenix.

This morning, it is a slow rise. The sun seems to take its time peeking over the horizon and chasing the shadows from the corners of my small, square room. Outside, a prayer is being recited over a loudspeaker.

The call to prayer has become familiar to me since my arrival here in Senegal, where 95 percent of the population practices the Islamic faith. The harmonious and soothing sound is comforting to my spirit as I roll off my inflatable mattress to salute the sun in my morning yoga and meditation ritual.

The stretch of reverse warrior, the bend of triangle pose, and the contractions of cat and cow are exactly what my body needs after the grueling 16-hour taxi ride yesterday back to Dakar from Saly, Mbour, the seaside town where I'd been based for my intensive dance training. This long day of travel has made my body feel stiff and tired after having spent so much time moving.

Today will be my last full day in Senegal. And, as I shift into each new yoga pose, I reflect on my journey so far.

I arrived here 11 days ago, thanks to a professional development grant from the University of California, Riverside, where I had just been hired to teach West African dance. Despite my credentials in dance, I felt compelled to visit the motherland to gain firsthand knowledge and education on the subjects of West African dance and culture. I felt this was the validation I needed to legitimize my teaching of this subject at the university level. Also, it satisfied a long-awaited dream of mine: to set foot on the land of my African ancestors.

Although I am African American and consider this my motherland, I have felt more foreign here than I could have imagined. Those around me most often speak Wolof or Mandig, native languages of the Senegalese people, which I don't understand. I have longed for home, although I am home in a sense. I have missed my children, my mother, and my husband, Jerome, all of whom were back in the United States. Despite these challenges, I am so grateful for this journey. Since arriving, I have learned so much, and today will be another important day in my education.

After my morning practice, I take my time dressing. I put on a tie-dyed, loose-fitting jumpsuit over my pink camouflage bikini. We will be traveling to Gorée Island today. Located about one mile off the coast of Dakar, this island is known for its role in the 15th- to 19th-century Atlantic slave trade. Despite (or perhaps because of) this dark history, it has become a popular tourist destination for both locals and foreigners. People go to tour the House of Slaves, the best preserved of the 28 slave houses that once dotted the island, and to swim in the azure blue waters.

As I emerge from my room, Triola – my friend, host, and guide in Dakar – is waiting. She rushes me out of the apartment. Her husband, Iba, is already outside waving down a taxi.

Triola tells me that she will not tour the slave house with me.

"I visited before when my mom came," she explains. "I don't need to go in again."

There is a song about Gorée that I have performed many times with my dance companies. The song is a lament for the atrocity of enslavement and a dedication to those Africans who left from that port. We often choose to sing it before dancing *Lamban*, even though it can be sung before many dances. We feel this is appropriate, given that Lamban is known as a healing dance. It is also a dance that thanks The Most High for music and for creating the *Jali*, the word for oral historians of West African communities located within the former Mali Empire. Lamban dates back to the 1500s, before the conquest of Africa and its people. Today, it is danced by members of the community, as well as the Jali themselves, who are still considered important members of Senegalese society. The Jali trade continues to thrive, and is passed down through the bloodline.

As we drive through the streets of Dakar, we are initially quiet. I think about my first day here, when I learned Senegal's traditional dance, *Sabar*.

Sabar originated from the Serer people, the third-largest ethnic group in the country. It is danced often and at many different occasions, from marriages to political gatherings. Sabar music is played with a sabar drum, which is hit with the hand and a stick. The dance includes quick turns, as well as jumps and rapid high kicks stylized by hip and thigh movements that require ample quadriceps strength. The ends of dance combinations are often punctuated by pelvic thrusts.

My teacher, "Pop," had taught me the basic five-step sequence from which all the other moves are based. Over the centuries, people have created many different variations. During the class, we'd danced elbow to elbow, cramped in Triola's living room. Nonetheless, I loved it. After that, I had headed to Saly, Mbour to continue my studies.

Triola and Iba want to know about my experience there.

"How were the rest of your dance classes?" they ask.

Gazing out the window of the taxi, I see a woman carrying a basket of sandals on her head. I am reminded of my sandal, which had broken while I was taking a class on the beachside. The sand had squished between my toes and made it more difficult to do jumps.

Triola chuckled as I described that day.

"I had to humble myself to learn *Koukou* again," I told her. Koukou is a celebration dance for the fishing harvest, and is a common rhythm encountered in African dance classes in the United States, as well as at events across West Africa.

"Koukou is one of the first dances I learned when I started studying and practicing West African dance," I continue. "I've studied it with many different African teachers and performed it many times."

"Well, It sounds like you learned more than just dance," Iba says, smiling.

"That's true," I reply. "Putting down my ego and listening to the ancestors opened me up to being a better student. It took away my arrogance so I could receive the ancient wisdom that my dance teacher, Aisha, was giving me. I learned so much in all our lessons, whether we were dancing outside on the beach or inside on a tile floor in stale air with no working fan."

"It sounds like dancing outside would have been more comfortable," Triola says. "Did you get to do that often?"

"Oh, yes!" I reply. "We would break into dance even while relaxing under a tree!"

I talked about the day when Aisha, her family, and I had watched

Aisha's two-year-old cousin, Imani, shimmy and shake in her new raffia skirt. Earlier in the week, Aisha had come to the compound with three colorful rice sacks. She'd shown me how to pull the horizontal threads out of the woven plastic bags, leaving vertical lines of brightly colored plastic string attached to the top band. In the end, we had made three skirts for me to take home and one for Imani to wear.

"They make great skirts for performing on stage," I tell Triola.

"You must show the skirts to me before you head back to Cali!" Triola says, obviously intrigued.

"I certainly will," I reply. "I tell you, we had a good time that day. They sang a 'call-out' song in the Sere language, and each woman danced when she heard her name. When little Imani was called up, she danced in her Easter-green skirt, and Aisha's two aunts and her cousins, Khady and Awa, were called to dance, too. When I heard my name, I was scared and reluctant."

"Why?" Iba asks.

"I did not want to look like a fool!" I respond.

"Oh girl, please!" Triola exclaims, "You are an awesome dancer!"

"It's different dancing in front of people who participate in the dance as part of their culture," I explain. "I don't want to be disrespectful of the culture by doing the wrong move to the wrong rhythm or moving the wrong body part in the wrong syncopation at the wrong time. Still, I answered with a few unsure steps, and we all laughed and continued to enjoy the cool breeze into the dusk."

"I am sure the family was glad to have you there," Iba says.

"Oh, yes," I say. "Before I left, one of Aisha's aunts gave me an outfit made by her tailor. It was a sheer, flower-patterned *buba* (blouse), with matching head wrap and light brown *lappa* (skirt). It was such a generous act of kindness."

As our taxi swerved through the morning traffic, I told my friends more about this sweet memory.

"At first, I didn't think it was for me. I said, 'Oh, this is nice!' and handed it back to her. But then she pushed it back to me!"

My story is interrupted as the taxi pops over a few potholes: *Bop badop bop badop bop bop*! It sounds like the break in one of the rhythms I've recently learned. The break is a signal from the drummers to the dancers that tells them to change, stop, or start a dance move. Triola, Iba, and I sit quietly for a few moments as the taxi makes its way over the uneven terrain.

When we're back on a smooth stretch of road, I continue, "The gift was unexpected, and I was honored, delighted, and taken aback. When I put the outfit on, it fit like a glove."

Aisha's aunt asked me to show the tailor, pointing me in the direction of the door to his workshop. As I walked over, the tailor stepped out. I posed a vogue or two. Then, I marched over to him, tossed my hands out side to side in Lamban fashion, and started dancing.

"What!" Triola exclaims. "You started dancing Lamban?!" Her face lights up with added interest.

"Yes, girl!" I reply. "And they all clapped and laughed with joy. Then, I got down on one knee, swung my head left and right like I'd done before in Lamban choreography, and tossed my hands up in gratitude toward the beaming tailor. He clapped, smiled, and said, 'Oh, good! You are good. Good dancer. Nice, nice!'"

"He's right; you are!" Iba adds.

"Thank you," I answer.

Recalling the last couple of weeks reminds me about the many powerful and beautiful moments I've experienced in Senegal, as well as how invaluable this trip has been for my understanding of West African dance. I would encourage anyone who studies African dance to visit the continent in order to better understand the context of why people do the dances.

In Senegal, I have learned, dancing is a part of life. In addition, I have never had the chance to immerse myself in African dance technique before. Being here, and having the chance to work with Senegalese teachers, has given me so much more than a 90-minute class taught in an air-conditioned studio in the United States ever could.

It's difficult to believe that the journey is almost over. I am in love with this land, and yet I feel ready to go home. I am excited to share what I have learned with my students, but I am sad to say goodbye to my gracious hosts and dance teachers. I am ready to see my family and my community, although I will miss the friends I've made here. These conflicting feelings are difficult to explain.

Although I do not plan to dance today, I consider this trip to Gorée Island a critical part of my education here. Gorée is a place I want to see for myself, not only because I have sung about it, but also because I know that this is one of the last places where my ancestors might have been before their forced entry into the *Ma'afa*, a Kiswahili term that means "terrible occurrence" or "great disaster," and refers to the Atlantic slave trade, as well as other events in what has come to be known as the African Holocaust. For the African American who performs traditional West African dance, Gorée is one place that represents the severing of the cultural right to learn the dances of their ancestors. I want to reconnect and reclaim my right.

When we arrive at the ferry terminal, a large crowd has already formed. Lines of people stream from the tall, thick metal doors attached to a massive, stone-walled industrial building. A large sign reads, "*Liaison Maritime Dakar-Gorée*" (Dakar-Gorée Maritime Link).

"I've never seen it so crowded," Triola tells me. "Ramadan is coming soon. They are probably getting in their last hoorah." During Ramadan, the Islamic holiday of reflection and fasting, Muslims spend time praying, reading the Quran, and often doing charity work.

There are three lines: one with young children in blue-and-white school uniforms, as well as one for men and one for women.

We move into our respective lines, doing our best to stay close to Iba. As we approach the entrance, there is a lot of pushing and shoving to get through the front gate. It's like an out-of-control rave, or a flash mob gone wrong. Iba grabs Triola's hand; Triola latches onto mine, and Iba gracefully squeezes us between the youth and through the doors.

"Wait here; I'm going to get our tickets," Iba says.

He disappears into the crowd and, a few minutes later, emerges with three tickets.

As we all board the ferry, guards remind the students again and again not to push and shove. Their excitement is causing a forward thrust in the lines that makes me feel uncomfortable and trapped. Once on the boat, we sit on benches in a room enclosed by plastic windows and a white metal roof. The students hustle and bustle between the seats.

As the boat begins its journey to the island, I step outside. I watch the dock on the mainland shrink as we move farther from the shore. Looking toward our destination, I see black bodies splashing around in the island waves and jumping off of a long pier into the water.

When we dock, Iba, Triola, and I wait for the majority of the crowd to disembark. We then make our way off the ferry and onto the island. Immediately, vendors and beggars approach us with their wares and palms exposed. We walk on, trying to avoid the eyes of a poor man in a wheelchair with one stump leg wrapped at the knee. Throughout my time here, as I have regularly come face to face with the poverty in Africa, dance has helped me stay focused on the beauty and power on this continent.

I am anxious to meet our tour guide, a middle-aged man named Abubacar, whom Triola knows. She catches a glimpse of him and waves him over. It's easy for me to remember the guide's name, as the drummer who accompanies my dance classes at UC Riverside has the same one. After introducing us, Triola flings her hands in the direction of the House of Slaves, sending us on our way. Then, she and Iba sit down in the doorway of the building across the walkway to wait for me.

As we approach the building, I read the sign above the entrance: "*Ministere de la Culture; Maison des Esclaves*" ("Ministry of Culture; House of Slaves"). Outside of the heavy, aqua-painted doors, I pause.

Stay strong! I say to myself, knowing this will be an emotional experience. I think of the *Doundounba* – the dance of the strong man or the dance of the warrior – and call on the strength of that dance to usher me past the threshold.

I am not alone with Abubacar on this tour. Two middle-aged men who look like tourists, with their sun hats and digital cameras, have joined us. Abubacar leads us to the left and into the first chamber. I take a deep breath and press "record" on my camera. I hang on every word as 400 years of history, cruelty, and devastation spew from his lips.

I document the cold rock walls, the damp floors, and the formerly blocked and locked windows that now allow slivers of light to creep into what were once dungeon cells. I hold it together, though disgusted by the once-disease-ridden quarters, each room with its own inhumane purpose. There is the feeding room, where Africans were fed beans with palm oil to fatten them up to an acceptable traveling weight. There is the weighting room, where Africans were weighed to determine whether they would be sent overseas. If they were not heavy enough, they were instead sold in exchange for trinkets and spirits. There is also the breeders' chamber, where slave owners kept boys as young as five years old.

The song about Gorée starts to play in my mind as I think of these children. Who among them could have been in the Jali bloodline? Being separated from the family to be used solely as reproducers was not only cruel: it also meant they wouldn't get a chance to receive the wisdom of their elders and carry on this sacred art and duty.

We walk through the virgins' cell, where young women were placed. These women were carefully guarded, because if they lost their virginity, they would be allowed to stay in Africa as domestic workers. I think of how much of their culture they missed by being sent to the Americas. They probably never got the opportunity to dance *Mandjani*, the dance of the young virgin girl. In my dance classes, I'd learned that to dance Mandjani is to accept a great honor. There are only two or three young ladies within a generation who are chosen to learn the dance and therefore to join the society of women called Mandjani. I wonder who among the young women kept in this cell might have become Mandjani, or were already Mandjani and carried the dance across the seas with them.

There are also the punishment rooms under the staircase, where Nelson Mandela had once entered and come out crying like a baby from empathy and disbelief that a man could survive being packed inside and sealed in the cold, dark enclosure with up to 15 other sufferers.

Finally, we reach the last room, where young virgins would wait, naked and linked together two by two. They were unable to move far because of the thirty-pound metal balls chained to their feet. Young ladies in this last room would sit in terror, knowing they would soon drag those metal balls down the hall toward the Door of No Return: the name for the last door that Africans on Gorée Island passed through before boarding the slave ships.

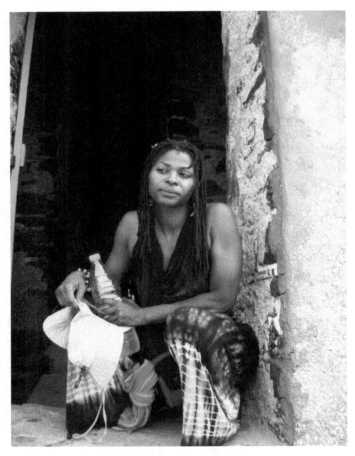

The author gazes out from the Door of No Return
Photo credit: Abubacar the tour guide

I stand in a place where my ancestors may have perished, suffered, and endured for my survival, and realize that a multitude of today's social dysfunctions were created right here. I intend to discuss this more with my West African dance students, feeling more compelled than ever to share this part of our global history.

Abubacar allows us to move through each room thoughtfully and slowly. He gives us time to soak in the moment and the history. By the time we proceed through the final hall and reach the Door of No Return. I am teary eyed. Standing there, I feel I have brought all of my ancestors with me: the bearers of the dances I so love today, from whom this incredible culture was stripped away as they arrived in the Americas.

For a moment, I stare out at the sea. The air is crisp and redeeming. The breeze is subtle as it whispers, *You are home*. I gracefully extend my arms to the left and then to the right. Then, I draw them across my body, hugging myself.

Yes, I am home, I reply.

"I suggest you visit the upper quarters, too," Abubacar says to me gently. "There are other artifacts there."

I head upstairs where rifles, shackles, trading pots, maps, and pictures are displayed beside informational plaques. Then, I progress to the downstairs artifact area. The walls are plastered with paintings and pictures of the mansion, memorial art, and photos of dignitaries who have visited, including Nelson Mandela, Bill Clinton, Pope John Paul II, Danny Glover, and Angela Davis. I am a little disappointed that they have not put President Obama's picture up yet, as I know he had visited Senegal a few years into his first term.

As I am leaving, I see a small book resting on a waist-high wooden pedestal. Its pages are filled with salutations and signatures. This is a way to leave my mark on this place: a way to say I have been here, brought my ancestors here, and proved that the name "The Door of No Return" is a lie. A sensation of contentment soothes my body as I sign the guest book: "I returned! Makeda Kumasi/Clydean Parker. *Sankofa!*" This last word is a Yoruba term meaning, "Go back and get it."

After touring the rest of the island, I reconnect with Triola and Iba, and we walk over to the rocky beachfront. We joke about diving off the tall rocks into the deep waters as we stroll amongst the cannons.

"I'll do it!" I proclaim.

I muster up the courage and strength of my ancestors as I remove my swimsuit cover-up, glasses, bracelets, camera pouch, and sandals. Barefoot, I brave the prickly rocks as they stab my soles.

Finally, I am standing by the side of the ledge in my pink bikini, watching as others make the jump themselves. I see a collage of moments in my mind: my family members jumping off a large slave ship, hoping to swim to shore in safety, yet knowing how unlikely that was; men and women taking the leap, thinking it better than an unknown fate on the other side of the world; and my ancestors being transported across the ocean, forced to dance on the decks for exercise. While dancing had been an integral and joyful part of their everyday lives before, now it was a way to survive.

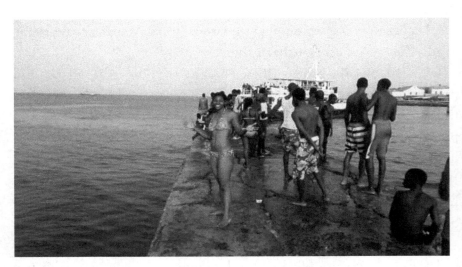

The author on Gorée Island, preparing to jump into the water
Photo credit: Triola Dulaney-Ndiaye

I think about how I will jump in their honor, and consider making a flying leap, arms wide open like a free bird expanding its wings for flight. Triola is ready to take a picture.

"Make sure you get the shot!" I yell to her.

"Okay!" she shouts back. "Give me a count so I know."

Looking over the edge, I cannot tell how high up I am. Perhaps two or three stories? Below me, fish are swimming in the water. Standing on top of the rocky pier, I am invigorated. I think of my ancestors, and how much I've learned since arriving. I am afire with new movements, new knowledge, and a rejuvenated spirit from the experience of learning in this place where the dances I love were born. A sense of gratitude arises in me for these new insights, as well as for the opportunity I have to share it with my students back home.

Dive! Just dive! I convince myself before counting off.

"One, two, three...!" I cry.

I leap off the rock and stretch out, ready to pencil dive into the sea. As my body splits the air around me, I feel totally free. Down I go, plunging into the cool, salty water. Yes, we have returned. Aséooooo!

Recommended resources:

Barnett, E. (2012, February 23). Senegal's Scenic Island Exposes Horrors of Slave Trade. Retrieved July 06, 2020, from https://www.cnn.com/2012/02/21/world/africa/goree-island-senegal/index.html

Charry, E. S. (2000). Mande Music: Traditional and Modern Music of the Maninka and Mandinka of Western Africa. Chicago, IL: University of Chicago Press.

Fieldstadt. (2017, November 22). The Most Heavily Muslim Countries on Earth. Retrieved July 06, 2020, from https://www.cbsnews.com/pictures/most-heavily-muslim-countries-on-earth/6/

Kästle, K. (1998). Senegal – Country Profile – Nations Online Project. Retrieved July 06, 2020, from https://www.nationsonline.org/oneworld/senegal.htm

Kumasi, M. (2016). 12 Days in Senegal: An Artist's Journey [Kindle]. Xlibris. Retrieved July 6, 2020, from amazon.com

WE 3 PRODUCTIONS (Producer). (2014, August 4). 12 Days in Senegal: An Artist's Journey [Video file]. Retrieved July 6, 2020, from https://www.youtube.com/watch?v=NembwrXUO84

Welsh-Asante, K. (2002). African Dance: An Artistic, Historical, and Philosophical Inquiry. Trenton, NJ: Africa World Press.

A MONTH IN MANILA

Kara Nepomuceno

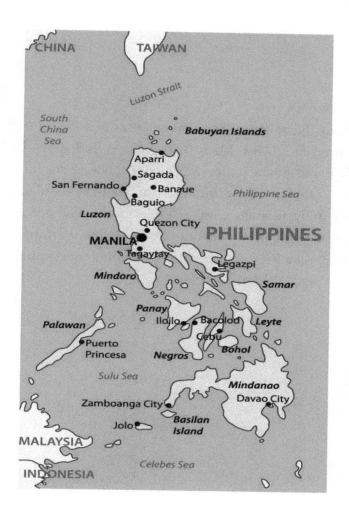

About the author: Kara Nepomuceno is a Shansi Fellow at Universitas Gadjah Mada in Yogyakarta, Indonesia. In 2019, while she was a senior at Oberlin College, she received a Shansi In-Asia Grant from Oberlin Shansi to travel to Manila and study *pangalay* dance. While in the Philippines, Kara worked with the AlunAlun Dance Circle performing arts group. Kara is a second-generation Filipina American raised in San Diego, California, USA.

I sighed and stretched my legs, which were starting to cramp after a two-hour cab ride through the metro area of Manila. This morning, my aunt and I were traveling from my grandmother's house to AlunAlun Dance Circle's studio, where I would train in the dance style *pangalay* for the next three weeks. As a member of the dance group, my aunt had helped me coordinate this opportunity.

My aunt had first seen AlunAlun during their performance at a human rights conference in 1990. Mesmerized by the artists' graceful rising and falling movements, she had begun taking weekly classes at their studio in the neighborhood of Marikina. Over the years, as she balanced her commitment to her growing family, she also began touring with the group in Vietnam, India, Cambodia, Myanmar, Laos, and Hong Kong.

Her direct connection to a pangalay dance group had inspired me to apply for a grant to further study this art form in the Philippines after learning the basics in the United States.

"Thanks again for supporting me with this, *Tita*," I said, using the word for "aunt" in Filipino. While my family members had grown up speaking English, a result of the US colonization of the country from 1898 to 1946, many of their conversations were a combination of Filipino (colloquially called Tagalog) and English. We call this mix "Taglish."

My aunt leaned over and reassured me, "I was happy to help you. I'm sure everyone at AlunAlun is looking forward to meeting you, too."

"Will you be dancing with us today?" I asked.

"I'm out of practice, but I think I might join in," she replied.

I nodded and began warming up my hands in anticipation, rolling my wrists in and out, and kneading my fingers.

We turned onto a street, and the driver pulled up to the curb to let us out. SUVs and motorbikes sped past us as we made our way along a row of gray cement buildings. Despite the area's muted appearance, I felt a rush of lightness and excitement. We were almost there!

Leaving the clamor of the road, we stepped tentatively past an iron-barred gate into the quiet interior of the AlunAlun Dance Circle studio.

It was a small, cozy space with large windows and glass doors that led to a veranda full of vibrant green plants. In some ways, the studio looked different from those I was used to. There were no mirrors, and my feet brushed against smooth stone rather than wood. Hats, masks, and fans – costumes for AlunAlun's shows – were hung around the room.

As we entered, members of the group smiled warmly and reached out to my aunt.

"It's good to see you, Mariel!" they said, welcoming her. She returned their smiles and laughed good-naturedly as she hugged each person. It felt like a reunion. The dancers were catching up and even exchanging small gifts.

"You're lucky to be here now," my aunt said to me after she'd greeted each person. "It's the first real practice of the year." People were just beginning to return to their normal schedules after the New Year's celebrations the previous week.

She then introduced me to the members of the group. Five people were in attendance that day. These dancers, men and women between the ages of 30 and 80 years old, were all professionals who held jobs in industries including health, education, and media. After some time socializing, we moved onto the tile floor to begin our warmup.

In silence, the dancers formed a circle. I followed along, watching carefully. Each member of AlunAlun took turns guiding the warmup, with leadership moving around the group. As one dancer demonstrated a step, the others would follow. As I began this experience with my new mentors, I reflected on my journey with this dance so far.

***

My exploration of pangalay began during a summer apprenticeship at the Samahan Filipino American Performing Arts and Education Center in my hometown of San Diego. This organization is dedicated to teaching and providing performances in Philippine dance and music. After having grown up training in ballet, I wanted to explore dance traditions that I thought would affirm my identity as a Filipina

American.

At this time, I knew little about my ancestry and the diverse history of the Philippines, but I felt Filipino dance might be a good place to start. With parents who had been raised in the cities of Manila and Angeles, I assumed I could perform anything from the 7,000-island archipelago. I had no idea about the artistic, demographic, and cultural differences between ethnolinguistic groups in different parts of the country.

Apprenticing at Samahan would quickly challenge my assumptions. I learned and watched many dances from the Philippines, some of which illuminated aspects of the country's history. Dances such as *tinikling* and *payong*, associated with the central Luzon region, had originated at the time when Spain had colonized the Philippine archipelago. This imposition had lasted 300 years, and led to the region becoming predominantly Catholic. It had also created a class of wealthy Tagalog families who worked for the Spanish state. In this way, many artistic traditions became representative of the nation that the Spanish would soon name after their monarch, King Philip II.

Other art forms, such as the *ciega* folk dance, depict old customs around courtship in the upper-middle class, and exemplify the Spanish version of the "ideal" Filipino: wealthy, well-educated, Catholic, and land-owning. Performing to the strumming of a guitar ensemble (which had also been introduced by the Spanish), women twirl in long, European-style dresses through several partnered and group dances. The men also wear Spanish-influenced clothing, typically sporting loose pants rolled up to the calf, a plain shirt, and a kerchief tied around their neck.

After the Spanish occupation ended, these dances developed into a folk canon: a series of dance suites performed and accepted as a representation of national culture. They now form a national narrative about Filipino identity.

At Samahan, I learned suites associated with indigenous groups who live in Cordilleras, a mountainous region north of Luzon; Muslim groups who live farther south in the region of Mindanao; and the predominantly Muslim Tausug, Yakan, and Sama communities in the Sulu Archipelago, a chain of islands in the southwestern part of the country. I gravitated most towards dances from the last area—and especially pangalay.

The first time I saw this dance, it looked so slow and fluid that time itself seemed suspended. As my instructor demonstrated for the class, his hands and arms decelerated, moving gracefully between each pose. His eyes focused gently on the tips of his fingers. As he came to the end of the dance, he uncurled his hands into a gesture with his palms upturned. His fingers were held together and curled back toward his wrist, his thumb thrust forward.

In that moment, a memory flickered. I recalled seeing my aunt in a similar pose, draped in a jewel-toned sash from shoulder to hip. She had posted the photo to our family's group chat years before, but I had forgotten its context. I messaged her later that I had begun learning the same dance.

"That's wonderful!" she wrote back. "Send me photos and videos of your next performance!"

The more I learned about pangalay, the more I appreciated it. My teachers at Samahan told me the dance focused on the curving and curling of fingers and palms, with performers often wearing long, metal fingernails to accentuate the shapes made by their hands. In class, I began to learn a rich movement vocabulary that seemed to reflect the beauty of the Philippine archipelago. Gestures represented ocean waves, a palm leaf, a gust of wind, or the flutter of a bird's wings.

As a slow but constantly moving dance, the practice made me feel deeply connected to my breath, my internal sensations, and my imagination. In class, I relaxed into the feeling of curving my arms and hands through the air, imagining the flowers and birds of the islands as I transitioned between each gesture. Each time I raised my arms and bent my knees, I saw myself dancing before a wide horizon of sand and water. As I glided slowly across the floor, I could be swaying on the sand or balancing on the bow of a long fishing boat. This dance, born in a community next to the sea, made me feel connected both to the San

Diego shoreline and to the Sulu Archipelago. While I had never been there, I imagined it was a region of vibrant blue seas and thriving wildlife.

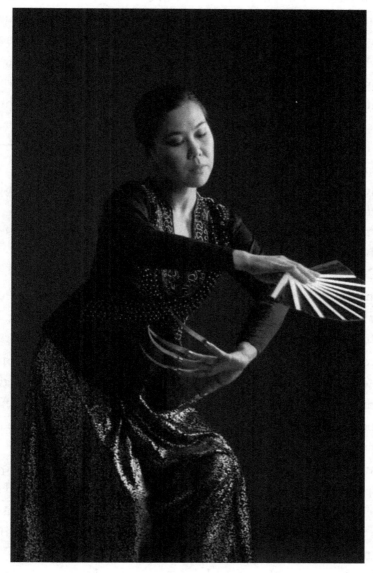

Nannette Matilac of AlunAlun Dance Circle performs Igal Kabkab (the Fan Dance) using pangalay movement vocabulary in a choreography by Ligaya Amilbangsa
Photo credit: Earthian Magazine and Medge Samblaceño-Olivares

As a slow but constantly moving dance, the practice made me feel deeply connected to my breath, my internal sensations, and my imagination. In class, I relaxed into the feeling of curving my arms and hands through the air, imagining the flowers and birds of the islands as I transitioned between each gesture. Each time I raised my arms and bent my knees, I saw myself dancing before a wide horizon of sand and water. As I glided slowly across the floor, I could be swaying on the sand or balancing on the bow of a long fishing boat. This dance, born in a community next to the sea, made me feel connected both to the San Diego shoreline and to the Sulu Archipelago. While I had never been there, I imagined it was a region of vibrant blue seas and thriving wildlife.

After our summer recital at Samahan, I emailed my aunt a video of my performance.

"I'm the one on the right!" I wrote, attaching a blurry clip of our ensemble piece.

"Congrats, Kara!" she wrote back. "What a thrill to see you doing the pangalay poses and gestures so recognizably. It reminds me of my teacher Ligaya Amilbangsa's classes with AlunAlun Dance Circle."

After that summer, I continued to practice, becoming more and more curious about what I could achieve in this art form. In the past, I had often felt anxious about how I looked. I had worried I did not fit the slim, delicate appearance that many expect of a ballet dancer. But this body type wasn't required in pangalay, and the sustained and deliberate motion of the dance provided me a sense of calm.

Pangalay was also easy to practice. While other dances required long spaces or special floors, I learned pangalay could be danced anywhere, even at home in your kitchen. Because the dance focuses on the curving motion of hands and arms, rather than the legs and feet, I didn't need a lot of space to rehearse.

One thing about the dance did give me pause, however. As a person of Tagalog and Ilokano descent, with a family who is still part of the majority-Catholic groups who live in Manila, I didn't have a link to the Tausug, Yakan, and Sama communities in which the dance originated.

I wanted to be respectful of these traditions and make sure that it was culturally appropriate for me to engage with them. I would need to learn more about pangalay's context, and figure out if there was a way for me to do this dance without reproducing harmful stereotypes.

From reading I'd done, I had learned that performers from outside Tausug, Yakan, and Sama communities sometimes made artistic choices that misrepresented those cultures. They might portray characters as stoic rather than expressive, or use dark lighting and smoke to create a feeling of mysticism. These choices unnecessarily exotified these groups.

With these thoughts in mind, I decided to apply for a grant to train further in pangalay. This is when I reached out to my aunt.

"Tita," I wrote to her, "I have really enjoyed learning pangalay at Samahan this summer, and I'd like to explore the dance further. What if I came to train with you and the AlunAlun Dance Circle?"

***

Now, several months later, I was beginning my first dance class in Manila.

Joy Cruz, who would later teach me private lessons, was among those in attendance. That day, she was wearing a loose t-shirt and long pants that rippled as she moved.

After the warmup, Joy explained more about the style of pangalay we would practice.

"It is called the Amilbangsa Instruction Method, or AIM," she said. "This form was named after its founder, Ligaya Amilbangsa, and it is based on her experiences and study of dance in the Sulu Archipelago."

I recognized the style, as it was the foundation of the choreographed dance I had learned at Samahan.

As we practiced that day, Joy took the lead in giving me gentle and specific instructions.

"Bend your knees more, and breathe slowly," she said, helping me to glide, rather than shuffle, across the floor. "Great, now repeat the movements on the other side for balance."

As I copied the improvisations of a senior member, I felt the shared breath of our small group. We moved together, fluidly and deliberately.

On the stone tiles of the one-room studio, we spiraled and sprang to the quick rhythms of a *kulintang* (a series of brass gongs that sit in a wooden stand) and the rush of the street outside.

"Break, *muna!*" someone said, after we'd been dancing for an hour.

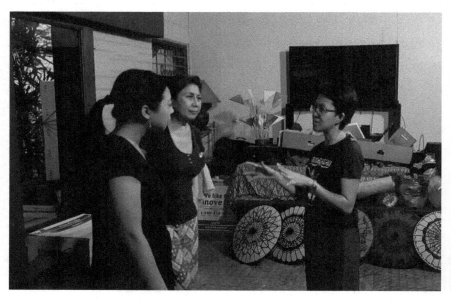

The author, her aunt Mariel Francisco, and Joy Cruz at the AlunAlun studio in Marikina, Philippines. Joy is explaining the first group lesson.
Photo credit: Thelma Padero

My aunt handed me a cup of water, and, as I raised it to my lips, I realized my lower back and arms felt sore. I had never danced so deliberately or in such a sustained way before. For the rest of the break, I stretched and chatted with the members of AlunAlun.

"Have you met Tita Ligaya yet?" Joy asked me.

"Not yet," I said, eyes widening. "Is she here?"

"Not today, as she's injured," Joy replied.

"Oh, I hope she's okay!" I said. "Could you tell me more about her?"

"She was raised here in Manila, but married a *Tausug datu*, a community leader," Joy replied. "Based on her experiences in Tausug communities in the 1970s, observing dance at social events and weddings, she broke the movements down into a codified form that would make the dance form accessible to more people. This became AIM, which she now teaches here in the city."

I nodded, appreciating the context. Pangalay was so much more complex than I'd first thought. The form I had learned at Samahan was not representative of the dance everywhere, but was instead Tita Ligaya's specific style, created from her personal history and experience. This had been a great way for me to get a grounding in the basics, as well as to explore what performers felt was essential to the dance.

"So there are many different ways to do pangalay?" I asked to confirm my understanding.

"That's one way to put it," my aunt answered. "What you learn with us is different from what you might see in Sulu, and younger generations have developed their own ways to dance, too."

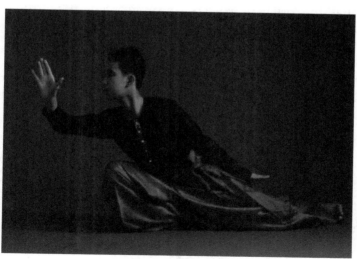

Jimo Angeles of AlunAlun Dance Circle demonstrates the kneeling and crouching stances that characterize pangalay male movements in the Amilbangsa Instructional Method
Photo credit: Earthian Magazine and Medge Samblaceño-Olivares

There is a lot of variation in the dance form, my aunt and Joy went on to explain. Dancers could bend their knees, flutter their fingers, and shake their shoulders in different ways. AlunAlun dancers, for instance, bent very low and aligned their breath with their motion. They also focused on making wavelike gestures with their hands rather than on the shoulder movements associated with newer styles.

"These variations are an important part of our practice," Joy explained. "As Tita Ligaya says, there is no 'correct' way to dance, although we believe some techniques are more beautiful than others." Her eyes sparkled as she gave me a teasing smile.

Later on, AlunAlun members and dance scholars would also show me videos of pangalay being danced in many different environments. Sometimes it was on the beach, and the movements mirrored the rolling waves. Other times, dancers performed on outdoor stages, in furnished tents, or in living rooms. While I'd known pangalay could be danced in many different settings in the United States, I hadn't known this was also true in the Sulu Archipelago. As it turned out, my romanticized notion that the original dancers only practiced in nature was not grounded in reality.

Furthermore, I learned pangalay is also practiced in Malaysia and Indonesia. In these countries, Tausug people are known as "Suluk." Both these names roughly translate to "people of the current" and refer to these communities' proximity to the ocean.

As I watched the dancers in many different urban and remote locations, I was inspired by their individuality, rather than their adherence to a codified form. They weren't reproducing a standardized style or trying to perform "authentically." Instead, they expressed artistry through their own distinct interpretations.

***

After that day at the AlunAlun studio, I continued to train via private lessons with Joy at my aunt's home in the Ayala Heights neighborhood of Manila.

During our first lesson, Joy gave me further context about the AIM warmup.

"This was created by Tita Ligaya to help novice dancers achieve the flexibility needed for pangalay," she told me as she showed me how to stretch my fingers back past my palms. We then stretched our fingers as far apart as possible while pushing our thumb and pointer finger together. This created a shape similar to the bird of paradise flower.

"It might hurt a bit at first," Joy told me. "You'll get used to it over time."

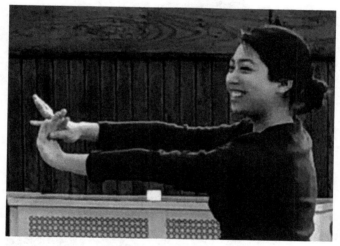

The author demonstrates the AIM hand stretch at Oberlin College
Photo credit: Jill Medina

She also helped me refine my steps in the AIM choreography of *linggisan*, which includes movements resembling seagulls flying, pecking, fishing, and scratching. In this dance, the performer also does other gestures that represent blooming flowers, swaying seaweed, a praying mantis, and crashing waves. There is no story involved – just themes – which makes it different from many other dance forms in Asia.

When I first started learning linggisan, I was traveling too much, stepping quickly back and forth across the floor.

"You don't have to go so far," Joy told me gently. "Also, I want you to try this movement with your arms."

Smiling, Joy demonstrated the shape. She lifted her arms out straight, creating a soft line just below her shoulder height. I took special notice of her flexibility, which made the shape possible. Her elbows, wrists, and hands were all slightly hyperextended.

"This will come with time," Joy assured me.

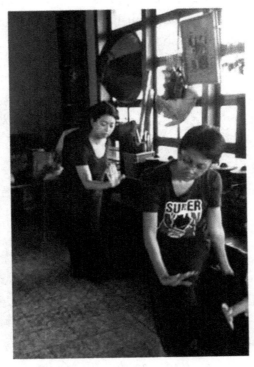

Joy Cruz (front) demonstrating AIM in the AlunAlun Dance Studio in Marikina, Philippines. In this movement, arms are extended in opposite directions. The dancer draws a figure eight with both arms as they sway from the front to the back of the body.
Photo credit: Mariel Francisco

I tried the move while applying Joy's feedback. Settling into the dance, I felt myself relax, feeling gratitude for this training opportunity with such an attentive mentor.

***

My three weeks in the Philippines flew by. On the day of my departure, AlunAlun was having a potluck party at Tita Ligaya's home. My aunt and I had come prepared for the occasion with the best fresh melon we could find. While I had met Tita Ligaya by this time, I had never been to her house. It felt like a special moment.

Before our shared meal, Tita Ligaya invited us to sit in a circle so she could demonstrate variations of a gesture she calls *kolek-kolek*. As we gathered around her, she began to show us a rolling motion of the hands that could be punctuated with a flick of the palms, or drawn out with a feathering of the fingers. We all tried to do it along with her.

After a few minutes of this group practice, Tita Ligaya came over to me. She watched carefully as I made the gestures with my hands, and made adjustments to the positions of my fingers when necessary. She paid special attention to my thumb, which needed to slide gracefully across the line where my fingers met my palms, as my hands slowly rotated outward. I was again reminded that these movements, which might look simple and slow at first glance, contain much more nuance and depth than one might assume.

Since Tita Ligaya knew that I would be leaving soon, and that I would be sharing this dance form with others, she encouraged me to practice these hand gestures whenever I could.

"You can do them on the flight home, on a bus, or on the streets of San Diego," she said. Then, she took a step back.

"It's time for your final exam," she said jokingly. "Let's see what you've learned during your visit. Show us linggisan!"

I hadn't known I would be asked to dance at this final celebration. Because I hadn't prepared anything, I would need to improvise with the steps I had learned over the past three weeks.

With my heart beating wildly, I went over to my bag and pulled out the stack of curved aluminum nails that Joy had gifted to me. Several members of AlunAlun moved to my side. They took my shaky hands in theirs and adjusted the ornaments to each finger.

"*Salamat po, salamat*," I said, thanking them as I flexed my hands slowly.

Joy and the other members of AlunAlun went to the front of the room and sat down, smiling warmly. As I walked to the opposite corner, my breath caught in my throat. I felt afraid to mess up, but I tried to remember that I had only just begun to learn about this style of dance, and that my audience was kind and rooting for me.

I paused, waiting for the music, and shifted my weight onto the balls of my feet. As the rhythm of the kulintang gong began, I lifted my right wrist in a curving line and slid my right foot forward. Then, I slowly repeated the movements on my left side, making my way to the center of the floor.

"Watch your shoulders," someone said, and I quickly lowered my tensed shoulders away from my ears.

Breathe, I thought, while trying not to look at myself sideways in the long, floor-to-ceiling mirror.

I focused on my senses. The air felt warm and humid, and my soles stuck slightly to the smooth wooden floor. After moving a bit stiffly through the basic steps, I felt reassured by a nod from my aunt. The kulintang then sped up, and I tried to remember the gestures that would depict different animals and plants. Focusing on the sway of a palm, or the flight of a seabird, I imagined my limbs transformed into branches, wings, and water. As I was a beginner, it was challenging to repeat every movement on the left and right, and I found myself going faster for fear I would bore the group.

"Slow down, slow down," I heard a voice say. I couldn't see who it belonged to, as I was focusing so intently on my fingers that everything behind my hands was a blur. I reluctantly slowed down, my thighs burning a little in protest. It took a lot of strength to move in such a sustained way.

My heart began to beat faster as I approached the most difficult sequence in the dance: one that would require the strength and flexibility I'd been working on since my arrival. I exhaled, crossing my arms and bending my torso forward. While continuing a wavelike motion with my hands, I extended my left leg in front of me and lowered myself to the floor by bending at the right knee. When I had gone low enough to sit on my heel, I rested for a moment, and then pulled my left leg back in and rose on both feet. Exhaling, I repeated the movement sequence on the other side.

I tried to make my transitions smooth, and wondered if I looked more relaxed than I felt. My hands were sweating, and I could feel the ornament on my little finger slowly slipping off.

I reminded myself to move thoughtfully and deliberately, trying to channel my inner calm and my connection to the ocean waves. This was my moment to show the members of AlunAlun how much I had appreciated this visit, as well as how my skills had improved thanks to their support.

Standing up with my knees still slightly bent, I began to walk slowly forward, shifting my weight from side to side. With each step, I turned my head toward my rising hand, which felt gentle yet strong, like waves that gradually erode a cliffside. As I reached the corner of the room, I dropped my arms slowly as the kulintang stopped.

I looked up to see the group smiling and rising from their seats on the floor.

"You passed!" my aunt said brightly, knowing the others would give me more tips for improvement before I left the celebration that evening. While I understood that I would need much more practice to skillfully dance pangalay, I still felt grateful for what I had been able to learn during just one month. With a sigh of relief, I followed her outside to the picnic table where our fresh melon was waiting.

***

After returning to college at Oberlin, I continued to train. One afternoon, when I was feeling empty and homesick after weeks of fast-paced work, I decided to practice pangalay in a second-floor dance studio.

Entering the room, I felt the warmth of the spring sunshine filtering in through the window. I raised my arms as I began to dance, making the swaying figure eight that Joy had taught me. Settling into the flow, I added in the hand motions I'd learned from Tita Ligaya. My fingers fanned outwards while my wrists rotated, creating circles in the light.

I slowed my movements further, relying on the rhythm of my breath to guide me. Painting my palms through the air, I found joy in the sensation of the breeze on my fingers. I imagined standing on the edge of the Pacific in the presence of the great ocean's exhale. Taking my time in this deliberate practice, I felt like a rising tide: expansive and ready for change.

Recommended resources:

Etnik Suluk Sandakan, T., & Etnik Suluk Sandakan, K. (Directors). (2009, August 24). *Suluk / Tausug Song ' Tiyula Itum '* [Video file]. Retrieved July 7, 2020, from https://www.youtube.com/watch?v=sRJj1cDH6Wc

Gaerlan, B. (1999). In the Court of the Sultan: Orientalism, Nationalism, and Modernity in Philippine and Filipino American Dance. *Journal of Asian American Studies, 2*(3), 251-287.

Quintero, D. A., & Anis Md Nor, M. (2016). The Curvilinear Ethnoaesthetic in Pangalay Dancing among the Suluk in Sabah, Malaysia. *Wacana Seni Journal of Arts Discourse, 15,* 1-25.

Stargazer Arts (Director). (2008, August 29). *Linggisan - Ligaya Fernando-Amilbangsa* [Video file]. Retrieved July 7, 2020, from https://www.youtube.com/watch?v=aafKF_KZx8A

MAKE ME PROUD, MS. COURTS

Courtney Celeste Spears

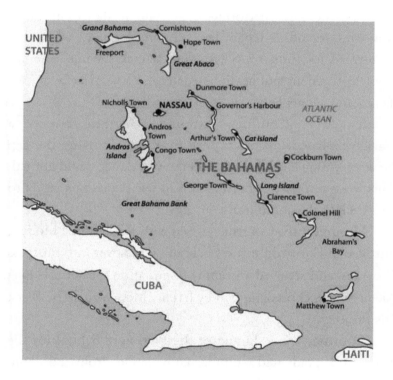

About the author: Courtney Celeste Spears is a professional dancer with the world-renowned Alvin Ailey American Dance Theatre. While growing up in Baltimore, Courtney frequently traveled to The Bahamas. Of Bahamian descent, and with family still residing in The Bahamas, she considers the country a second home.

Courtney has performed and taught dance in many countries, including Japan, France, and Germany, where she performed for former US President Barack Obama. She has been featured in publications such as *Vogue*, *The New York Times*, and *Vanity Fair*.

In 2017, Courtney co-founded ArtSea Dance, a Caribbean-based organization dedicated to bridging the gap between young local dancers and the vast dance world abroad. This work is a part of her mission to use dance as a vessel to give back to the community.

Most recently, Courtney signed with Wilhelmina Models, enrolled in Harvard Business School's Crossover into Business Program, and received an Emmy nomination for her role in *A Mother's Rite*, choreographed by Jeremy McQueen's The Black Iris Project.

Courtney is an alumna of the Baltimore School for the Arts, and graduated summa cum laude from Fordham University with a Bachelor of Fine Arts in dance and a degree in communications.

I woke up to the *zzzzzz* of my phone vibrating under my pillow. Opening one eye, I saw that it was still dark outside.

Who would be calling me this early? I wondered.

Looking at the caller ID, I saw it was Terri Wright, my dear friend and fellow company member at Ailey 2, the junior company of Alvin Ailey. I knew this call must be important. Today was a big day for us, after all. Terri, the other company members, and I would be traveling from New York City to Nassau, The Bahamas, as part of our international tour.

I picked up the phone.

"Hello?" I said, feeling groggy.

"Where are you?" Terri asked. "Are you meeting us on the bus?"

I pulled the phone away from my face and looked at the time: 6:45 a.m. Panic shot through me like a lightning bolt, jolting all the sleepiness out of my system. I'd set my alarm for 4 a.m.! Why hadn't my alarm gone off?! The entire company was about to leave the studio to get on our bus to the airport, and I was still in bed.

"I'm meeting you at the airport," I told Terri, trying to play it cool. "Gabriel and I are on our way. Don't worry!"

I hung up and immediately sprinted down the hall to wake up my best friend, then-roommate, and fellow company member, Gabriel Hyman. For some reason, his alarm hadn't gone off either. As Gabriel realized what was happening, he too panicked. Luckily, we had packed the night before. We quickly threw on clothes, brushed our teeth, and called an Uber.

Twenty minutes later, as we sped toward the airport, I felt as if I had a steel weight in my stomach. It was my second year with the company, and this part of the tour had been arranged *specifically because of me*. How would it look if I were late to the airport? And what would happen if I missed the flight?

I thought about how upset our artistic director would be, and then my thoughts shifted to my grandmother. What would it be like for her to show up at the Nassau airport and see all the company members but me? How would that make her feel? We were very close, and I looked up to her immensely. I did not want to let her down.

I stared at the clock in the Uber and prayed that we wouldn't hit any traffic. We were lucky, and arrived at the airport just in time to meet everyone else at check-in.

As we went through security, boarded the plane, and sat down in our seats, I remained in a slight state of shock. Because of this, the significance of what was about to happen did not hit me until two hours later when I looked out my window and saw that we were officially over The Bahamas' waters.

From the time I was a child, I have traveled to The Bahamas a minimum of three times each year, and sometimes up to eight. I have spent every holiday, spring break, and summer on the islands, so by now I could tell when the plane crossed from US territory to that of The Bahamas.

As I looked down, the view of Florida was slowly replaced by the dark blue ocean. As the plane approached The Bahamas, the color of the water changed to an ombre of lighter blues, interrupted only by tiny white- and peach-colored island droplets. The scene grew increasingly beautiful as more and more of The Bahamas' 700 islands came into view. The one I could most easily identify was the island of Eleuthera, a thin strip of land that's about a mile wide and 110 miles long. Watching this scene from the window was something I always looked forward to.

While so much of this journey seemed familiar, this time there was something very different: I was going as a member of Alvin Ailey. My company members and I were on the way to *my spot, my home, my sanctuary.* This trip was the culmination of the work we had done as a dance company, as well as the effort that my community in The Bahamas had put in. Once they had heard that I was in the company, my grandmother, friends, and family had become relentless about finding a way to bring Ailey 2 to the islands.

As the plane touched down in Nassau, I thought of my grandfather, Frank Theodore Sweeting, who was still alive at the time. He was, as Bahamians say, "born bred Bahamian." He was my giant: a tall, dark-chocolate man whose smile was contagious. He'd played baseball for

The Bahamas National Team and led them to victory, earning him a spot in The Bahamas Baseball Hall of Fame. He was self educated and self employed as a taxi cab driver. This was how he'd managed to put all of his kids through college, keep a home that we all treasured, travel to New York for family vacations, and even have money to put in my pocket every time I came home. He was, and still is, my hero.

"Go and make me proud, Ms. Courts," he would tell me. "Always put God first, and go make me proud."

And here I was with my entire dance company, about to dance for my Bahamian community and to introduce Ailey to the country I so loved. Furthermore, I knew that my mother, my Pops (stepdad), my father, and my brothers had all flown to Nassau to see the performance that night. This was the ultimate proud moment. Overwhelmed with gratitude and excitement, I began to cry.

As we exited the airport with our bags in hand, we were met by my grandmother, Andrea Sweeting; the director of the National Dance School of The Bahamas, Mr. Robert Bain, and Mr. Bain's right-hand woman, Ms. Renee Davies. These were the people who had taken the lead on bringing us to Nassau, which had been no easy task. To secure the funding, my grandmother, Mr. Bain, and Ms. Davies had written letters to the government and to businesses. They'd also worked with local vendors to secure discounted hotel rooms, airfare, and the work permits required for us to perform in the country. They'd even found a gorgeous place for us to perform: a big theatre at the Atlantis Resort on Paradise Island.

My grandmother was waiting for me outside with a huge smile and her arms open, ready to give me a giant hug. I was thrilled to see her.

"We're here, Grammy!" I said, embracing her. My grandmother or my grandfather had always picked me and my family up from the airport. When I was a child, I would run out to see them while my mom waited for our bags.

"We have some very special things planned for you," my grandmother told me.

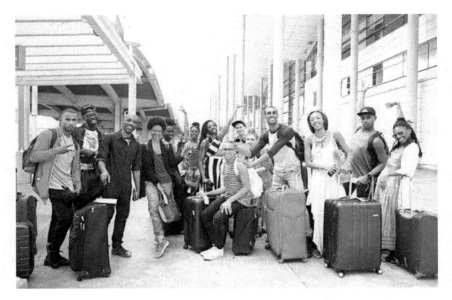

Members of Ailey 2 pose for a photo at Lynden Pindling International Airport in Nassau
Photo credit: The Nassau Guardian

I had been expecting this, trusting that my community would welcome my colleagues in the typical warm way we are known for. If you ever visit The Bahamas with a Bahamian – or even just as a tourist without any connections – you'll notice how inclusive the community is. We Bahamians love to rep where we're from, and we want to show you a good time, feed you, and tell you about the culture.

"The island has been buzzing with excitement," my grandmother said.

I felt myself blush. That year, I happened to be the Ailey 2 poster girl, so pictures of me dancing were plastered all over The Bahamas on the ads for the show.

"When everyone heard there was a Bahamaian in the company and that you were the woman on the poster, they were thrilled," my grandmother informed me.

Tickets had sold out, she added, and my mom was receiving tons of messages from her friends.

"Dede, is this *your* Courtney performing?" they asked. "Is she really coming to Nassau? If so, I have to see this! I have to see her dance."

"Yes, that's her!" my mom would reply. "That's our girl."

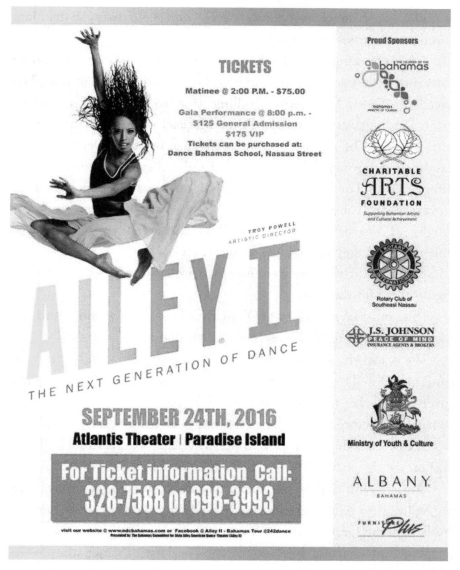

The author featured on one of Alvin Ailey's posters in 2016
Photo courtesy of the Alvin Ailey Foundation and Eduardo Patino
(NYC)

The upcoming event was even more exciting because of its rarity. Despite the fact that it is less than a three-hour flight to New York City from the islands, dance doesn't travel to The Bahamas in the way that it could. Most dance companies never come, and many Bahamians haven't seen professional dance.

After checking into the hotel, we prepared to visit the former Governor General of The Bahamas and treasured Bahamian icon, Her Excellency Dame Marguerite Pindling. Her late husband, Sir Lynden Oscar Pindling, was the former Prime Minister of The Bahamas for 25 years and led The Bahamas to independence in 1973. Her Excellency has dined with royalty all over the world and dedicated her life to serving the people of The Bahamas. She is our queen, and being invited to Government House to meet her in person was an honor and true privilege. I'd never been there myself, and the chance to go for the first time with my company felt like a huge honor.

When we arrived, we were met by her guards, who shared with us the protocol for the visit.

"She must be addressed as 'Your Excellency,'" they said. "And you cannot touch her until she reaches out her hand to touch you."

We'd also chosen our outfits based on protocol. Men had to wear pants and closed-toe shoes, while women needed to have their shoulders covered and be modestly dressed. We had received all of these instructions before flying to The Bahamas so we could pack accordingly.

"Now introducing Her Excellency Dame Marguerite Pindling," said one of the guards.

Anticipation built in me as Her Excellency walked gracefully down the hallway in a billowing, colorful dress. As she approached us, her eyes landed on my grandmother. Within a few moments, the two were hugging and chatting like old friends—because, in fact, they were! Although I didn't know it at the time, they had sat next to each other at St. Agnes Anglican Parish, one of the largest Anglican churches on the island, every Sunday for years.

"Who is your grandmother, again?" my colleagues jokingly asked me, wondering how she was so close with Her Excellency.

That moment was a testament to how small and intimate the island is. This exceedingly poised royal icon was also a mother, a grandmother, and active churchgoer. A sense of love and community filled the space.

Her Excellency welcomed us all into a sitting room, where we gathered in a circle.

"I heard there's a Bahamian in this group," she said.

"It's me," I said, feeling nervous to be addressed by such an incredible woman.

"Who is your family?" she asked. In The Bahamas, this is a common question. Because communities are so tightly knit, you often discover that you know members of someone's family when you hear their last name.

"Well, that's my grandmother next to you," I replied, feeling proud and delighted at being able to provide the connection. My grandmother started giggling, and so did Her Excellency. They looked at each other and then both looked at me. We all smiled.

***

Later that evening, we headed straight from the Government House to a welcome party held at the home of a family friend and my grandmother's fellow breast cancer survivor, Virginia Hall Campbell. Virginia's home is beautiful, and also has a stunning view: it sits right on Lake Cunningham.

As we walked into her home, we were greeted by Mr. Bain, my grandmother, Ms. Renee, my brothers, Asa and Aaron Cary, my parents, and some of Mr. Bain's students.

They welcomed us into a room full of tables covered in authentic Bahamian *Androsia*, a local fabric that feels like a thicker version of linen and comes in blue, green, pink, and orange hues. On top of the tables was a smorgasbord of traditional foods.

Before eating, Mrs. Virginia said a quick prayer. This is how everything, from meals to sports games, is traditionally opened. Then it was on to the meal!

Food is a core of many aspects of Bahamian culture. The first stop I make whenever I arrive in Nassau is for a cold Kalik or Sands (two local Bahamian beers) and one of our signature cultural foods: conch salad, specifically at the conch stand in Gambier Village.

To prepare conch salad, the local chefs remove the bright pink conch meat from the shell. They then chop it up right on the spot and add lots of ingredients, including tomatoes, onion, goat pepper, green peppers, orange juice, lime juice, and even fruit if you want a tropical conch salad. All of the juices and ingredients are overflowing from the rim of the bowl. It's absolutely delicious, and it's not pretentious. You eat conch salad out of a plastic bag with a spoon at conch stands stationed around the island. It's messy, packed with flavor, and – in my opinion – one of the best meals you'll ever have in your life!

"Y'all are in for a treat," I told Terri, Gabriel, and the others.

Mrs. Campbell had the conch salad presented in tiny little bowls, which was an elegant twist on a very casual meal.

As Terri took her first bite, her eyes brightened.

"Oh my goodness," she said. "This is delicious."

She went back for seconds, as did the rest of us.

As I sat with my friends, watching them enjoy the conch salad, conch fritters, macaroni and cheese, guava duff, johnny cake, and other local dishes, I was still in awe. I couldn't believe I was sharing my Bahamian traditions with these people I so cared about. The foods my colleagues were eating were the local dishes my grandmother had cooked for me over the years and that I had shared with my family over holidays, birthdays, and other celebrations. This is my version of "soul food."

As I sat and ate with my colleagues from Ailey, we talked about the arts in The Bahamas.

"How is the dance culture over here?" Terri leaned over and asked. "What's it like?"

"Dancing and the arts in general are truly loved in The Bahamas," I replied. "You can see how much we love dancing in celebrations like Junkanoo, which features tons of West African dance. Junkanoo is a street festival and celebration that goes from 10 p.m. on Christmas night all the way until Boxing Day afternoon. During the event, drummers, dancers, and musicians in elaborate costumes and floats make two full laps around Bay Street in Nassau's main downtown area. Afterward, there is dancing and performing all night long. The performers' costumes are spectacular! People are covered from head to toe in beads, feathers, bells, crepe paper, and glitter. There are massive floats, and the sound of instruments like sheepskin drums and cowbells echo through the downtown area."

Since this was one of my favorite annual events in The Bahamas, and as I had watched many friends and family members prepare to dance in the event, I had a lot to say.

"For some dancers here, dancing in Junkanoo is their only form of dance training," I said. "I often wonder if they realize how rich that training is! Many people start learning from a young age, and they develop a lot of stamina. Junkanoo is rooted in West African history, which means that much of the dance movement and choreography has its origins in grounded, traditional West African steps. Performing West African dance to live music for almost a full day takes so much endurance! Also, all these dancers are taught to understand intricate parts of musicality, so they have the ability to improvise to live music and find their place if their dancing is ever interrupted by a loud crowd, blowing winds, or anything else going on around them. Because of all this, The Bahamas is full of promising young dancers."

Terri nodded along as we talked.

"How about modern dance or ballet?" she asked. "With some training, I bet a lot of these performers would be great additions to those types of dance companies here or abroad."

"It's a funny thing," I replied. "Even though we love the arts, dancing isn't respected as a viable career option. Parents want their children to be successful, so they encourage them to go into more streamlined careers, such as becoming a lawyer or a doctor. Sometimes, when I tell people here that I'm a professional dancer, they ask me what my *real* job is. They still have a hard time believing that I make money dancing, that I went to college for it, or that working as a dancer gives me a consistent paycheck, benefits, and health insurance."

Once we all had food, Mr. Bain stood up to formally greet us.

"Welcome, everyone," he said. "We are so happy you are all here. There are many students at the National Dance School who are excited to see you. They've never watched anything like this live. When Courtney texted me to say you'd landed, I felt emotional. It's a culmination of the work we've done to bring you here, and I know it will inspire our community."

My grandmother and Mrs. Campbell also said a few words. Shortly thereafter, my mom stood up to speak, as well. I could see she was trying not to let her emotions overwhelm her: she was fighting to hold back tears, and her voice shook slightly.

"Thank you all from the bottom of my heart for being here," she said. "You can't imagine how much this means to me."

My mother, D'Andrea Cary, is my everything, including my connection to The Bahamas. Born and raised in Nassau, she had moved to the United States for college, where she met my father, Tyrone Spears. I was blessed that she had supported my dreams, even if she did not understand them. Like most Bahamians, my mother had pursued a more stable career. She had decided to become an accountant, and still loves the work to this day. When I had told her that I wanted to be a dancer, however, she had allowed me to pursue this goal. She'd had no idea what a career in professional dance looked like, but she had taken on my dream as her own.

While supporting me through my dance classes and other aspects of my childhood in Baltimore, she had also made sure I knew my culture and heritage. We would speak to my family in The Bahamas multiple times per month, thus staying connected to the pulse of what was happening on the island. On our frequent trips to the islands, we always attended church services at St. Agnes Anglican Parish with my grandparents. This is where my cousins and I were baptized, as well as where my grandparents, parents, and uncles were all married. In November 2018, we also buried my grandfather there. The traditions and values of my Bahamian family thus also felt like my own, even if I spent much of my time in the United States.

After several hours at the party, we headed back to the hotel. Before falling asleep that night, I texted my parents.

"Don't forget to text me where you're sitting in the audience!" I wrote. This was our tradition. They would tell me exactly where they were seated so I would know where to wave during a bow.

***

I started the next day with a prayer.

Dear God, thank you for having us here. Thank you for bringing my dance family here. I pray that you use us to be vessels of your love, greatness, and power. May today be an unbelievable one. Amen.

First thing that morning was the tech rehearsal, which would be our first introduction to the theater. As we entered the large, gorgeous space, one of the hotel managers informed us that the theater hadn't seen a live act in more than 20 years. Despite having a full proscenium and a stage, it was only being used to show movies. I felt sad hearing that, knowing that this could be such an incredible space for the performing arts. Even so, being able to breathe life into this stage – even if it was just for this one performance – felt like something special.

The show, we were told, had sold out. I couldn't wait for the community to see our performance. At Ailey, we have many different dance pieces that we choose from for each event. Tonight, we would dance "Something Tangible" by Ray Mercer, "Gemeos" by Jamar Roberts, and "In and Out" by Jean Emile.

Still on the stage, we then took company class, during which ballet and modern dance movements help us warm up before a performance. After that, we headed to the dressing rooms.

Waiting for the show to begin that night, I was anxious and nervous. I'm always a little nervous before I dance in front of an audience, mainly because I care so deeply about my work. This moment, however, felt particularly important. I wanted this performance for my

69

community to be spectacular.

As soon as I stepped on the stage, however, my nerves were replaced by pure presence. People are often surprised to hear that members of Ailey rehearse six to seven hours a day. When they ask why we practice so much, I tell them it's so that we can enjoy the stage. When you are well rehearsed, you can lose yourself in a performance.

During the show that night, I was grateful for all our hours of rehearsals. As I moved, I felt complete bliss, enjoying the dance and the sense of connection I felt with my people in the audience. My island had come to support me, to support us, and to support the Alvin Ailey legacy, which Ailey himself had said is about "bringing dance back to the people." As I danced through the pieces, my mind was quiet. It was just me on the stage with my entire Bahamian community and God watching.

When the performance came to an end, I looked out into the crowd. As usual, I saw my Pops, Andrew Cary, stand up first. He always made a point to rise and start clapping before everyone else at the end of the performance. With his arms raised high in the air, he exuded pride for me. I also caught sight of my father, whose eyes were filled with tears. He always gets emotional at my performances, seeing his little girl all grown up and following her dreams.

Finally, my eyes landed on my mother. The look of immense gratitude on her face will never leave me. I knew whatever I was feeling must have been magnified many times within her. This was a huge, full-circle moment for both of us.

There at Atlantis, we were just 20 minutes from my mother's childhood home. In a way, I felt like I'd grown up there, too. In the United States, I had always been focused on school and dance, rather than play. When we went to The Bahamas, I got to be a kid. I like to joke that every scar I have is because of the adventures I had with my family there: we used to climb trees, jump over walls, and race all around the neighborhood.

My mom had often expressed her concern that I wouldn't feel connected to The Bahamas despite our frequent visits. Well, here I was.

And I did. I was bringing my two worlds together, and it was an honor and a joy far beyond what I could have imagined.

After our bow, we headed out to greet the audience members. As we emerged, we were met by a huge crowd. Looking out at everyone's faces, I was particularly struck by the wide-eyed stares of the children, who looked at us like we were aliens. I was confused for a moment until I remembered Mr. Bain's speech from the welcome event: these kids had never seen a dancer live on a theater stage, let alone a performer emerge from backstage after a show. I hugged them all and thanked them so much for coming, making sure to ask them questions about why they loved to dance, which dance school they attended, and what they liked about the performance. I wanted to let them know that I believed their experience was important and how overwhelmingly grateful I was that they had come.

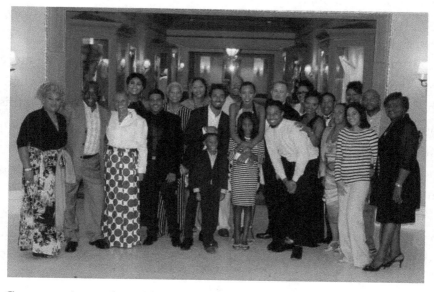

Courtney (center) and her Bahamian family outside of the Atlantis Theater post performance
Photo credit: Robert Bain

After spending time with the children, I noticed my grandmother standing nearby. She was waiting for me with open arms and the biggest smile.

"Grammy, we did it," I said. "What did you think?"

"I absolutely loved it," she responded. "My goodness, you all were so beautiful."

She then held up the program.

"Have you seen this yet?" she asked me.

"No," I said. "Why?"

She flipped to the section where companies typically placed their ads. Instead of ads, however, there were messages to me.

"See these letters of support?" she said, turning the pages. "People are so proud of you and the work that you and your colleagues have done. They purchased this space in the program to show you how much they appreciate you coming here."

As I was looking through the sweet messages, Mr. Bain approached me and gave me a hug.

"You've started something here," he said. "We can't stop it. We need to keep it going."

It was clear that Mr. Bain was referring to bringing more professional art experiences to The Bahamas, and I knew he was right. The Ailey dancers shouldn't be the only professional dancers this community had the chance to see in Nassau. Similarly, young Bahamian dancers deserved the opportunity to work with top talent from abroad and to learn of opportunities in the arts. There's only so much you can dream about if you don't see it for yourself.

I felt a deep sense of excitement. I'd never thought that my purpose to give back to the world could combine my two favorite aspects of life – dance and The Bahamas – but here was an opportunity to do just that.

***

Within eight months, I had co-founded ArtSea Dance with Asa Cary, my big brother, whose efficient, stern, and steadfast nature balances my creativity and imagination. ArtSea focuses on weekend-long conventions that support young artists in the Caribbean in cultivating their talent through dance classes, informational sessions, and paid performance opportunities at places such as Albany Bahamas, an exclusive resort on the western tip of the island, and Create Serendipity, a leading event production company in The Bahamas founded by my aunt, Megan Minus. Our goal is for students to develop a better understanding of the vast dance world abroad by learning from professionals in genres such as ballet, modern, jazz, contemporary, floor barre, and musical theater.

Today, four years later, ArtSea Dance is supported by many of the same people who helped with Ailey 2's first trip to The Bahamas. My grandmother, Mrs. Renee, and Mr. Bain are critical players, and we use the same sponsors who helped with logistics on our first trip. Furthermore, many more of my family members and friends have become volunteers. Myrkeeva Johnson, one of Mr. Bain's students whom I met at Mrs. Campbell's home, has worked with me on many projects. As I've developed relationships and worked in new ways with people I've known my entire life, building ArtSea has not merely felt like growing a business. It's felt like growing a family.

Together, we've raised in excess of $60,000 to put on workshops for more than 250 Caribbean students. Faculty members who come from Alvin Ailey, Broadway shows like *Hamilton* and *King Kong*, and other notable performing arts companies teach at these events, which are held at the prestigious Windsor Academy. And, while we cover instructors' flights, hotel stays, and food, they donate their time because they believe in our vision. Dance is truly the catalyst behind this effort. It inspires us to work together and to lift each other up.

While I never could have imagined co-founding a business in The Bahamas, I am so grateful that dancing and my community in the United States and in Nassau have made it possible. Through a shared vision and passion, we have come together to improve access to dance education and show our youth that they can do anything they put their minds to.

Since Covid-19, our audience has expanded beyond just The Bahamas. I'm excited for the future of dance in the Caribbean, and I am dedicated to doing my part. No matter how far I travel or how big my dreams grow, I'm most certain that this experience in Nassau was the catalyst for my own purpose. My values and my destiny are all wrapped in my Bahamian culture. As I think about the future of this project, I can hear my grandfather's voice, just as I did when landing in the Bahamas with Ailey 2: "Put God first, and go make me proud, Ms. Courts..."

Recommended resources:

Alvin Ailey American Dance Theater. (2020). Retrieved July 06, 2020, from https://www.alvinailey.org/

ArtSea. (2017). Retrieved July 06, 2020, from https://www.artseadance.org/

The Charitable Arts Foundation. (n.d.). Retrieved July 06, 2020, from https://www.thecharitableartsfoundation.com/   (ArtSea Dance Founding Sponsor)

Nassau Bahamas Chapter of The Links, Incorporated. (n.d.). Retrieved July 06, 2020, from https://salinksinc.org/   (ArtSea Dance Founding Sponsor)

PART 2: FINDING COMMUNITY

"Dance felt like my all-access pass to new conversations and friendships."
—Damilare Adeyeri,
from his Dance Adventures story, "Trying on a New Hat"

As I read the line above, I found myself nodding, remembering a spring night in the south of France. It was before the days of Uber, so I'd ordered a taxi to take me to a swing dance far out in the countryside. I hadn't considered how I would get home. Instead, I had trusted that I would make friends, and that one of them would give me a ride back to the city.

I was right and then some. I got a ride back to my hotel, as well as a late-night city tour and an open invitation to stay with the local dancers whenever I came to town.

The next day, as I shared what had happened with my non-dancing companions, they were stunned. They couldn't believe I'd made friends so quickly. When I tell this story to other dancers, however, they aren't surprised at all. People like me, Damilare, and the other authors in this chapter know how quickly dancing can create a sense of connection.

When we dance, we enjoy shared experiences of play, creation, and adventure with others, and this creates a bond. In this chapter, we celebrate that connection, which may last for the duration of a song or an entire lifetime. Whenever and wherever we dance, we can have this experience of community.

THE CARNIVAL CHRONICLES

Melaina Spitzer

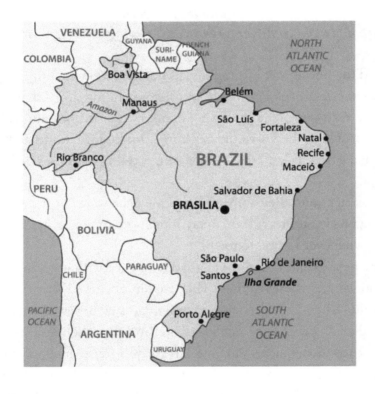

About the author: Melaina Spitzer is a dancer, leadership consultant, and certified coach devoted to helping people and organizations transform. She specializes in conflict resolution, change management, and leadership development. In her current role as a consulting partner for The Ken Blanchard Companies, she designs and delivers trainings for global leaders. Her keynote, *Building Resilience in Times of Crisis*, has provided tools for more than 2,200 public servants during the COVID-19 pandemic.

Melaina is also the founder of her own coaching and training company, through which she has worked with more than 1,500 leaders globally.

During her seven years living in South America, Melaina worked as a peacebuilder, human rights advocate, and reporter for the BBC and NPR. After returning to the United States, she served as the founding director of the travel company Dance Adventures from 2015 to 2018. In partnership with Megan Taylor Morrison, she designed and co-led trips across the globe, further witnessing how dance can build community and transform lives.

Melaina is fluent in Spanish and Portuguese, and loves dancing Argentine tango, Cuban rueda de casino, and Brazilian dança de salão. She holds a bachelor's in history of divided societies from Brown University and completed a master's in peace, conflict, and security as a Rotary World Peace Fellow in Argentina. You can learn more about Melaina at www.melainaspitzer.com and connect with her on Linkedin.

In Melaina's story, some names and identifying details have been changed to protect the privacy of individuals and organizations.

"*Olha, aí vem a Rainha!*" someone shouted over the deafening sound of the steel drums. "Look—here comes the Queen!"

The woman who entered the room immediately caught my attention. Her muscular legs seemed to move at the speed of hummingbird wings as she executed the triple steps of Brazil's national dance, samba. This powerful woman effortlessly shimmied and undulated her hips to the beat of the drums.

Seeing her, the drummers smiled, playfully shouted praise, and danced toward her as if she had ensnared them in an invisible web. Everyone else in the massive, brightly lit warehouse seemed to pause for a moment in reverence before letting their own feet go wild once again.

The woman, Adriana Carioca, held a coveted title: she was the newly crowned "*Rainha* (pronounced *hi-EEN-ya*) *da bateria*" ("Queen of the Drums") for one of Rio de Janeiro's premier samba schools, Felizes da Vida. One of 70 samba schools in the city, Felizes da Vida was known for bringing satire and humor to many of its performances.

The Queen of the Drums plays a critical role in each samba school. She is responsible for inspiring the school's drum corps to perform at their highest level, rallying the crowd, and performing the traditional *samba no pé*, a solo dance with intricate footwork done at breakneck speed. Contestants for this position were chosen based on "their looks, samba skills, and charisma."[1]

It was difficult not to stare. Not only was Adriana an amazing dancer, but she was already wearing part of her beautiful costume—or *fantasia* in Portuguese—for our upcoming show. During rehearsals, it is typical for performers to practice in the parts of their costume that may be tricky to dance in. In this case, Adriana was wearing a massive, blue-feathered headdress with elaborate peacock plumes that splayed out so far it appeared they could brush the ceiling.

She also sported an embroidered gold bikini top, cut-off shorts

---

[1] Grudgings, S. (2009, February 18). Life Not All a Carnival for Rio's Drum Queens. Retrieved July 12, 2020, from https://www.reuters.com/article/us-brazil-carnival-queen-idUSTRE51H4GS20090218

(which would be swapped for gold bikini bottoms at showtime), and shockingly high heels. As she sashayed around the floor, I wondered how she could walk, let alone dance.

The moment was interrupted by the voice of our director, shouting, "*Vamos galera–a dançar!*" ("Come on, people, let's dance!")

I brought my attention back to the choreography. After all, I had a job to do! In just a week, I would be performing as part of Felizes da Vida's ensemble for Rio de Janeiro's world-famous Carnival parade. My teammates and I would dance around the school's float while Adriana sparkled from the top.

I knew this wasn't just something to do for fun. It was a serious commitment. The fervor of pride and allegiance at each samba school is intense. Many *cariocas* (locals from Rio) identify themselves as *belonging* to their samba school. This means they are extremely loyal, like some people are to sports teams. Performers for each school relate to their teammates as close comrades, or even family.

As a white North American who had been living in Brazil for just over a year, I felt honored to have been warmly welcomed into the community and given the chance to take part in what is arguably Brazil's most iconic event. To show my respect for the culture and my teammates, I knew it was critical to treat this opportunity with the utmost care. I had been training hard, trying to learn as much as possible from my teachers about both Brazilian dance and the history and significance of Carnival.

Typically, performers at samba schools spend long hours rehearsing nearly year round, and their practices intensify around Brazil's summer season each year. Carnival's samba parade is competitive in nature, with different divisions for samba schools (think major and minor leagues, but with many more tiers). The goal for these samba schools is to make it to the highest level – the *Grupo Especial* (Special Group) – and then to win the competition.

During the parade, each samba school is allotted 75 minutes for its procession. Teams receive scores in 10 categories: their float, their "flow and spirit," their costumes, and more.[2] Points are deducted if the procession goes under or over the permitted time, and judges watch carefully, ready to lower scores when they see mistakes. If there are significant flaws, the school can even be demoted to a lower division in the rankings. Attention to detail is therefore critical.

Each school's routine is done to the original samba song they create for the event (another component of their overall score), which is composed by famous Brazilian musicians and songwriters and then performed by the samba school's own drum corps. The lyrics to Felizes da Vida's song this year paid tribute to the Lapa neighborhood, which is the historical center of samba and the heart of Rio de Janeiro's dance scene. It compared Lapa to a shining star.

Since its inception, Felizes da Vida had been working its way up the competition ranks. After getting the top score in Group B in 2012, they had been bumped up to Group A, the level just below Grupo Especial. If the team did well this year, it could mean an ascent to the highest level of competition. Knowing so much was on the line, we had been training for months, memorizing choreography and the lyrics to our school's samba song in hopes of becoming champions of our Carnival category.

***

In 2012, I'd moved to Rio de Janeiro with a plan to split my time between working as a radio journalist for NPR and for a social responsibility program with indigenous communities in the Atlantic Forest. Not long after I arrived, however, I began moonlighting in a third, unofficial role.

Each night after work, I took a hot, crowded, 45-minute bus bus ride to a tiny, sweaty studio in Lapa. There, I fed my heart and soul dancing with a *forró* (pronounced *foh-HO*) dance troupe. This dance style

---

2 Carnival Parades in Rio: Samba Parade. (n.d.). Retrieved July 12, 2020, from https://www.riocarnaval.org/samba-parade/parades-in-rio

from Northeast Brazil has become popular across the country. Forró is common at social gatherings, especially during *Festa Junina* (June festival), when Brazilians come together in large groups to eat, drink, and dance. This event is one of the largest festivals in the country, second only to Carnival.[3]

I'd fallen in love with this dance style and found out about the school while exploring the city's nightlife. In Rio, music pulses through the streets. There are fantastic parties every evening where you can find live music, as well as talented dancers and musicians who put non-professional dabblers like me to shame. After a few weeks of exploring various venues, I'd discovered my two favorite places to go.

On Monday nights, I would head to *Pedra do Sal* (Salt Rock), a giant, black volcanic rock that marks one of Rio de Janeiro's birthplaces of samba. In the heart of the Port Region, Pedra do Sal is known for its "historic importance as a *quilombo*, a home to the descendants of enslaved Africans brought to Brazil."[4] My fellow dancers had told me that nearby, Tia Ciata, a priestess of the Afro-Brazilian religion *Candomblé*, used to host parties. There, the Brazilian composer Pixinguinha and his contemporaries had developed modern samba music, which had its origins in *samba de roda*, a musical style brought to Rio from the Brazilian state of Bahia and recognized by UNESCO as part of Brazil's cultural heritage.[5]

In this neighborhood, the cobblestone streets were punctuated with steps that provided the perfect, elevated location for a band. People

---

[3] Brown, S. (2018, April 15). 10 Things to Know about Festa Junina in Brazil. Retrieved July 12, 2020, from https://theculturetrip.com/south-america/brazil/articles/10-things-to-know-about-festa-junina-in-brazil/

[4] McLoughlin, B. (2015, December 18). Pedra do Sal Quilombo Celebrates Ten Years with Procession and Bid at World Heritage Status. Retrieved July 12, 2020, from https://www.rioonwatch.org/?p=25826

[5] The Story of Samba at the Dawn of Modern Brazil: Roots of the Samba. (n.d.). Retrieved July 14, 2020, from https://afropop.org/samba-stories/2-roots-of-the-samba.html

of all ages would gather around a *roda de samba* (samba circle), a group of five to 15 musicians jamming out to their favorite samba songs.[6]

As the night unfolded, crowds would pour into the square. People would spill beer on the cobblestones as they moved in time to the infectious rhythms, dancing away their worries to the sound of the drums, tambourines, guitars, and the *cavaquinho*, a traditional Brazilian ukulele.

Wednesday nights were for dancing forró at the Centro Cultural Carioca, a cultural center in the heart of the city. Forró music is fun and fast. Songs almost always include the rhythmic sound of the metal triangle accompanied by the *zazumba* (an Afro-Brazilian drum), and an accordion or *rabeca* (a type of fiddle descended from the medieval rebec). The music was made popular by Luis Ganzaga, a Brazilian singer, songwriter, and poet who became one of his country's most influential 20th-century musicians.

The first time I went to the Centro Cultural Carioca was on one of Rio's infamous 40 °C (104 °F) summer nights. As I approached, I saw young people overflowing from the venue out onto the street as the syncopated bass beat of the zazumba lured me in.

The band was stationed to the right of the balcony, which spanned the entirety of the front of the room and overlooked the historic Praça Tiradentes square. It was lucky the windows were flung open and the fans on full blast, since the room was packed with sweaty twentysomethings.

During a particularly fast song, I was lucky enough to get swept up by a masterful *forrozeiro* (forró dancer). In a flash, we were moving in circles of light-footed bliss. Quick spins, hip pops, playful footwork, and the power of centrifugal force had me laughing, panting, and smiling

---

[6] Sims, S. (2018, September 08). Women Move from Samba's Sidelines to the Center of the Circle. Retrieved July 15, 2020, from https://www.nytimes.com/2018/09/08/world/americas/women-samba-musicians.html#:~:text=Step%20up%20to%20a%20traditional,%2C%20a%20cavaquinho%2C%20a%20drum.

from ear to ear. By the time the dance was over, I was totally dizzy—and completely hooked. I asked my dance partner where I could learn more, and he referred me to a well-known studio in the heart of Lapa.

Forró would become my happy place. I began attending dance classes at the school, where I heard about the opportunity to support Felizes da Vida in their Carnival performance. Felizes de Vida hoped that featuring a forró number – and therefore paying homage to the diverse cultures that make up the fabric of Brazilian music and dance – would help distinguish the school from its competitors. As one of the leading academies in the area for forró, our school was their top pick. I quickly agreed to participate. Now, months later, we were almost ready for the big show.

***

When I'd attended Carnival as a spectator the year before, I'd learned that it is so much more than a party, a show, or a parade. This annual event represents an intersection of politics, pride, community, artistry, and celebration. While some schools focus on showing off Brazil's unique cultures, other schools use Carnival as an opportunity to take a stand on current events impacting their community. Schools often use their songs, costumes, and sets to send political and environmental messages to the crowds lining the bleachers of the Sambódromo, a stadium created especially for the Carnival parade.

These performances can have a chilling effect. I remember how my jaw had dropped as I watched one group of performers emerge in elaborate costumes, dressed as birds whose feathers were covered in black oil. Row after row of swans danced solemnly past me, flanked by a river made of long swaths of shining, black, undulating cloth. Behind them was a float designed to look like an oil rig. It included giant drills that pulsed up and down, artificial flames, and workers doing acrobatics as they spun and did backflips off the machinery. Finally came a second float complete with a golden car, a larger-than-life-size golden pencil, and a gold dollar sign suspended in air.

This samba school had chosen to take a stand on an issue that was politically dividing the region: a bitter battle was ongoing between the State of Rio de Janeiro and other inland states over control of offshore oil rigs.[7] If the proceeds of oil exploration came to the State of Rio, the school was saying, there would be great benefits to infrastructure, health, and education. If control of proceeds from the rigs ended up in the hands of another state, however, there could be mismanagement—including massive oil spills.

This was indeed an ominous performance for Brazil. Five years later, in 2019, oil would wash up on the shores of at least 11 Brazilian states including Rio de Janeiro, requiring the removal of at least 4,000 tons of crude. While studies would eventually conclude that the oil had not originated from Brazil's oil rigs, the event was devastating for the people and animals inhabiting the 720 beaches, rivers, and mangrove swamps that were impacted.[8] In Carnival that year, that samba school had proven that no topic was too controversial for center stage.

***

After the final few intense weeks of training with my teammates, it was again the night of the Carnival Parade. This time, I was part of the show! My hands shook with anticipation as I attempted to apply my makeup while bearing up under the weight of my flashy orange-and-blue-plumed headdress. I could not believe I was about to have the

---

[7] Associated Press Reporter. (2013, February 11). "The Greatest Party on Earth": Rio Carnival Reaches Its Breathtaking Climax as Thousands of Scantily-Clad Samba Dancers Gyrate through the Streets in an Explosion of Music and Colour. Retrieved July 12, 2020, from https://www.dailymail.co.uk/news/article-2276859/Rio-Carnival-2013-photos-The-greatest-Earth-reaches-climax.html

[8] Associated Press Reporter. (2019, November 23). Oil from Brazil Spill Washes up in Rio de Janeiro State. Retrieved July 12, 2020, from https://apnews.com/a06be2b53da0499c8dd6c8c5543c0e08; Brazil Environment: Clean-Up on Beaches Affected by Oil Spill. (2019, October 20). Retrieved July 12, 2020, from https://www.bbc.com/news/world-latin-america-50113383

privilege of joining in one of the most meaningful events in Brazil.

To say I was anxious is an understatement. I wanted to do well not only to support the school, but to make sure my presence was a contribution to this cultural event. My heart pounded as I thought about the huge crowds and TV cameras that would be analyzing our every move.

There was also a more immediate problem: no one knew where our costumes had gone! In Rio de Janeiro, significant value is placed on maintaining a relaxed and carefree lifestyle. "*Deixa tranquilo*," (loosely, "Be chill") and, "*Relaxa!*" ("Relax!") were two of the phrases I heard often from my carioca friends. This was one of the elements I loved most about living in Brazil; however, it sometimes became an issue when there were deadlines.

For our Carnival performance, the timeliness of costume completion was essential. Luckily, Adriana's full outfit had arrived. In addition, the leaders' ensembles – overalls with long-sleeved white shirts – had come on time. Still, the other ladies and I were waiting for ours. We had only our headdresses and shoes, with nothing matching to wear in between them. And while some samba school performers were intentionally clad in nothing but body paint and glitter, this was *not* our plan.

As we continued to get ready at the studio, our contacts in the costume department kept assuring us that our outfits would be finished. After several hours, however, we were informed that they were not yet ready and would need to be delivered directly to the Sambódromo. Our director suggested we wear the bare minimum to the stadium so we could put the costumes on over our clothes. I chose a bright blue sports bra to match my headdress, and tiny gray shorts, hoping they wouldn't be too visible underneath. My teammates and I then jumped on the metro.

As we made our way to the Sambódromo, we mentally prepared for the huge crowds and the physical stamina it would take to complete our task. Our intense rehearsals had readied us for this incredible workout in the heat of Rio's summer nights.

After exiting the metro and walking for what seemed like an eternity, we arrived at the entrance to the famed stadium. With music blaring and colorful floats towering above us, I saw some of the most incredible artistry I had ever witnessed. Women donned petticoats that extended their twirling skirts at least six feet in any direction. Men suited up in animal costumes twice their size, and performers entered on stilts, soaring above us like giants. Emotion welled up in me: a combination of reverence, gratitude, adrenaline, and pride in my dance team. But I also couldn't ignore the nagging anxiety in my chest. Would our costumes be ready?

We watched from a distance as our director made several calls and his face grew more and more somber. His expression shifted from anxiety to disappointment, and finally to desperation. It wasn't looking good. At last, he approached the group and delivered the news we had all been dreading. There would be no costumes.

For a moment, we all stood staring at each other in shock. After so much hard work, though, my teammates were unwilling to give up. Defiantly, one of the men in the group unclipped his overalls, pulled off his shirt, and handed it to his dance partner. She looked at him knowingly, and in one fell swoop, the shirt was over her head. On her petite frame, it went down to her mid-thigh. It obviously didn't match her headdress and shoes, but that didn't matter.

Within seconds, all of the other men were pulling off their own shirts and handing them to their partners. I turned to my lead, Pedro, a sweet, bespectacled man in his early twenties. He looked at me nervously as we both realized that he was already shirtless under his overalls. That part of his ensemble had never arrived.

What could we do? I would never be allowed on the pitch without a costume. But Pedro had an idea. He scoured the crowd until his eyes landed on a heavyset man nearby with one unexpectedly precious asset: a white t-shirt. While it didn't perfectly match the ones the others were wearing, it was good enough! In a heartbeat, Pedro had disappeared from my side, sprinting across the pavement. I watched in amazement as he approached the man and began speaking quietly to him. The man nodded, and I saw a pensive look on his face. He shook his head no, and I thought for sure he had declined Pedro's request.

Just as my heart began to sink, something totally unexpected happened. The man began to smile. He tore off his v-neck and handed it to Pedro. The man now stood shirtless in the street, waving as Pedro sprinted back in my direction. Tears of gratitude welled up in my eyes for Pedro and his ingenuity, and for this stranger's act of service. It was the first—and only—time in my life when I would be overwhelmed with appreciation for being handed a sweaty shirt off a stranger's back. I threw it on and was ready to rumble!

My dance troupe excitedly approached the entrance. It was the moment we had all been waiting for, and there was no way we were going to allow this hiccup to inhibit our performance. We were so excited for our choreography that showcased the incredible tradition of forró at an event typically dedicated to samba.

When we reached the gates, I could see immediately that there was a problem. Security was scanning us dubiously, and two guards began whispering to each other. Then one of them approached our director.

"I'm sorry, man," he said. "If you don't have costumes, you can't perform."

Our director stood up straight, his frame suddenly energized in a way that made him look far taller than he was.

"Unless you have the Director of the *Bateria* (drum corps) come down here right now and tell me we can't dance, we *will* be dancing," he said. His eyes beamed with unequivocal pride and defiance. He had worked tirelessly to create this choreography. For our director, *we* were his star of Lapa. I could see in that moment that there was no way we could be prevented from performing. We were a unified community, committed to providing our contribution – our art – to this incredible spectacle.

Tension filled the air as everyone watched the two men glare at each other in silence. The security guard towered over our director, who stood firm. I could see that he would not back down—not now, and not if they had to carry him off the grounds.

That moment felt like an eternity. Would we be able to perform? Or would our dreams be crushed by the failure of our own samba school to complete and deliver our costumes? Finally, the security guard broke the stare, averting his eyes in embarrassment.

"Tá bom! Pode passar!" he yelled over the cacophony of drums. ("It's all right! You can pass!") Our troupe erupted in applause. Pedro and I jumped up and down and hugged each other.

We stepped onto the promenade in the gleaming lights of the spectacle and began to dance. We had made it. During the 75 incredible minutes that followed, it didn't matter that we weren't perfectly matched or that I was wearing a misfit t-shirt. Our individuality melted away into the unified, beating heart of the crowd.

As we executed our choreography, I spotted Adriana Carioca, our Queen of the Drums, atop one of the floats. She looked utterly majestic, emanating bliss as she danced samba no pé. We were all here together, and nothing in the world could extinguish the joy created by the celebratory union of art and community in that moment. We were samba and forró, Brazilians and foreigners, united by the power of dance.

Recommended resources:

Arôxa, J. (n.d.). Jaime Arôxa. Retrieved July 07, 2020, from https://jaimearoxa.com/

Baila Mundo (Director). (2018, January 21). *Baila Mundo - Jaime Arôxa e Robertinha Stephanie (Oficina do Samba Verão 2018)* [Video file]. Retrieved July 7, 2020, from https://www.youtube.com/watch?v=-xoSQI8_57c

Canal YouDance (Poster). (2012, October 7). *Felipe Barbosa, Gilberto Paixão e Marinho Braz com a família do forró* [Video file]. Retrieved July 7, 2020, from https://www.youtube.com/watch?v=T5Wir0vheS8

Cia Marinho Braz. [Portuguese only]. (n.d.). Retrieved July 07, 2020, from https://www.facebook.com/ciadedancamarinhobraz/

CroqueteFilmes (Poster). (2014, February 22). *Caprichosos de Pilares - Carnaval 2014 (Videoclipe Oficial)* [Video file]. Retrieved July 7, 2020, from https://www.youtube.com/watch?v=82vALpdSStA

De Oliveira, Jimmy. [Portuguese only]. (2017). Casa do Jimmy. Retrieved July 07, 2020, from http://www.casadojimmy.com.br/

Forró de Domingo (Director). (2014, July 1). *Forro de Domingo Festival 2014 - Valmir & Juzinha - Stuttgart, Alemanha* [Video file]. Retrieved July 7, 2020, from https://www.youtube.com/watch?v=c33sqgUUJKg

Renata Pecanha. [Portuguese only]. (2020). Retrieved July 08, 2020, from http://renatapecanha.com.br/portal/

Rosa, G. (Director). (2012, January 3). *Roda de Samba Jimmy de Oliveira e Suellen Violante* [Video file]. Retrieved July 7, 2020, from https://www.youtube.com/watch?v=Y8xcdISAqHM

SBKZ Media (Poster). (2019, November 3). *Renata Pecanha + Jorge Pires @ China Brazilian Zouk Congress 2019* [Video file]. Retrieved July 7, 2020, from https://www.youtube.com/watch?v=wb6ha7Fyt_o

TRYING ON A NEW HAT

Damilare Adeyeri

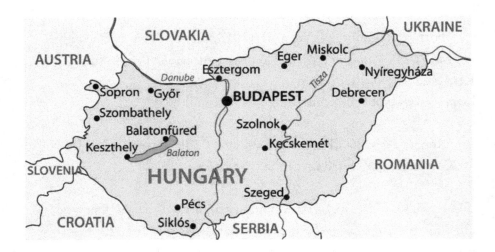

About the author: Damilare Adeyeri grew up in Nigeria, where he was immersed in the music and dance of Yoruba culture: Gbedu and Alujo rhythms, Batá drumming and dancing, and much more. From 2013 to 2015, Damilare traveled through Norway, France, Hungary, and the United Kingdom studying dance traditions as part of his master's degree in dance knowledge, practice, and heritage. He currently resides in Ann Arbor, where he is an international student and scholar advisor at the University of Michigan. Damilare is also a passionate salsa and bachata dancer, teacher, and performer, as well as a Zumba® instructor.

As I entered the school gymnasium, I was met by a chorus of fiddles, rhythmic stomping, and clapping. The space was packed with men and women engaged in lively conversation. At the center of the room, 50 couples danced to songs played by two violinists and a double bassist. The gymnasium had become a space for this *táncház* (literally translated as "dance house"), a Hungarian folk dance and social event.

I'd dressed for the occasion that night, making sure my outfit would be appropriate for this new experience. I'd donned a multi-colored, long-sleeved shirt tucked into black trousers, and a black hat. I'd chosen what to wear – and especially my hat – because it was similar to the style of the Roma men from Transylvania whom I'd met. I quickly made my way through the crowd, looking for the familiar faces of my graduate school classmates.

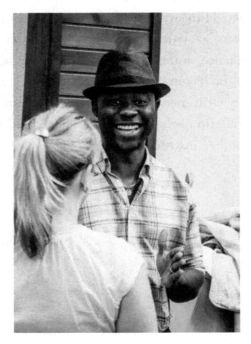

Damilare, just after arriving at the táncház in Szeged, Hungary
Photo credit: Department of Ethnology and Cultural Anthropology,
University of Szeged, Hungary

Although I'd known what to expect, I was still nervous. I had only lived in Hungary for three months, and I was still very new to the culture. Moreover, I stood out! In a part of the world where most people are white, there was no one else who looked like me. So far, this had only evoked appreciation and curiosity from local dancers.

"Where are you from?" people would ask me politely during social dance events. "What interests you about our dance? How did you learn it?"

I was once even asked these questions for an ethnographic documentary about the transmission of Hungarian cultural heritage in society. The researcher had noticed me dancing at a local event, and was intrigued since I looked distinctly different from the others.

Dance felt like my all-access pass to new conversations and friendships, and I had no reason to believe tonight would be different. Still, I wanted to be respectful of this culture's traditions. The Hungarian dances were different from the dances I'd learned growing up in Nigeria, but no less wonderful. I had great respect for the artists I'd met so far, and wanted them to know how much I appreciated their work.

*****

My journey into the world of Hungarian dances started as a result of working through a two-year Erasmus Mundus Master of Arts degree program called Choreomundus. The program was a partnership between four European universities, and focused on dance knowledge, practice, and heritage. I was one of 18 people from 15 different countries who had recently arrived in Szeged, Hungary. We'd come to continue our Choreomundus studies at one of the partner universities, the University of Szeged, for our third semester of the program. My colleagues and I had become close friends over the last year and a half of our program.

Csaba Varga, a Hungarian member of our cohort, played an especially important role on this leg of the journey. He had grown up in Kalotaszeg, Transylvania, and was like an honorary, additional professor who was deeply knowledgeable about many dances from the Transylvanian region.

Tall, fair-skinned, and slender, Csaba had a warm and unassuming look. He was a man of few words, but once you got to know him, he would engage you in fascinating conversation. I loved to hear him talk about the many Transylvanian folk dances that he knew, and especially the *Kalotaszegi Legényes* (lad's dance), which was his specialty.

While Transylvania is today a part of Romania, it was once part of the Kingdom of Hungary. Many Hungarians still live in the area, where a plethora of art forms were born before political lines divided the region into two different countries.

Our time in Szeged included a research course called, "From Field to Archives." The course focused on documenting Hungarian folk dances for the purpose of comparing past and present versions, as well for cultural preservation.

The minimum dance requirement for this course was to learn the basics of *csárdás*, a traditional Hungarian folk dance; however, I also fell in love with a dance called *mezőségi korcsos* the first time I saw it.

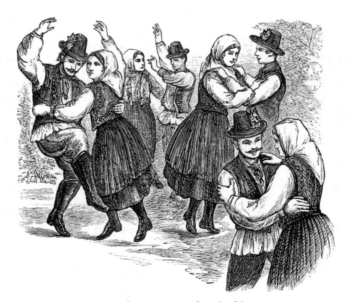

A depiction of csárdás
Photo credit: Wikimedia Commons

During one of our class rehearsals, Csaba started teaching us embellishments to the csárdás with moves borrowed from *korcsos,* a traditional Transylvanian men's solo dance from the Mezőség region of Hungary and a subtype of the *legényes* dances.

"The Romanian name for korcsos is *târnăveană*," Csaba told us. "That's what the local Hungarians and Romanians who still live in Transylvania call the dance. Târnăveană means, 'named after the Târnava River.'"

I was intrigued by the percussive nature of the embellishments.

"Would you teach me more korcsos?" I asked Csaba at the end of class that day.

"Sure!" he said. "I'm happy to do that if you want to learn!"

I was so excited! As a drummer, I was drawn to this dance that incorporated percussive sounds through clapping, slapping your legs, and stomping. These embellishments aligned with the music, allowing the dancer to express himself in several distinct ways.

Csaba and I agreed to meet occasionally outside of our group csárdás rehearsals so that I could learn and practice korcsos.

During our first meeting, Csaba taught me the beginning of a korcsos choreography that included various traditional moves. While korcsos dancers and musicians traditionally improvise off of one another, this requires an advanced level of knowledge and years of practice. Choreography was a way to make this dance accessible to me as a beginner. Still, it was a challenge. The choreography was fast—so fast that if I missed one clap or slap, it was difficult to get back on track.

As I messed up time and time again, learning this dance became more than a hobby: it became a mission.

I'm going to conquer this dance, I thought. Always up for a challenge and eager to learn about this culture through movement, I felt inspired and invigorated. At the end of every rehearsal, I recorded myself dancing. I watched those videos religiously in between sessions, going over each of the moves carefully.

It took about six weeks for us to work through the choreography and for me to become comfortable with the movements. One day, after

I had performed the whole dance perfectly during our session, the normally reserved Csaba cracked a smile.

"You know this now," he told me.

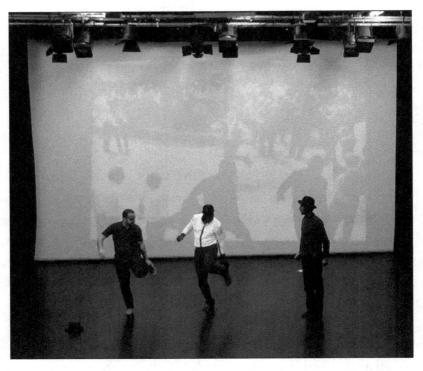

From left to right, Csaba Varga, Damilare Adeyeri, and Valér Bedő dance legényes in the Michaelis Theatre at Roehampton University in London. Behind them, a movie is playing that shows Hungarians doing the same dance long ago.
Photo credit: Damilare Adeyeri

After several weeks of preparation in the "From Field to Archives" course, we were ready for the final seminar. Eight Hungarian community members from the village of Vişea (or "Visa" if spelled in Hungarian) in the Mezőség region of Transylvania were coming to share their knowledge of Hungarian folk dances with us. We would work with them to document these dances for cultural preservation purposes.

Our professors chose community members from within

Transylvania, since it is a historically important area. Throughout history, Transylvania has been occupied by many different people. The Daco-Romans, Habsburgs (Austrians), Turks, Hungarians, and Romanians have all called this region home at one point or another. Ultimately, the Battle of Transylvania during World War I led to Transylvania becoming a part of present-day Romania.

The village of Vişea is unique because Hungarian and Romanian people live together there. In other parts of Transylvania, you most often find exclusively Hungarian or Romanian populations.

Our professors wanted to find people whose style of dance had been well preserved over the years. These villagers had been doing folk dances before the political borders were formed. In Vişea, you don't hear the same debates about whether cultural dance traditions are Hungarian or Romanian as you do in other communities.

"There are arguments about this elsewhere," Csaba told me one day. "I had always heard the Romanian Roma were mostly the musicians and the Hungarians were the dancers. I'm not sure anyone knows for sure."

During the villagers' visit, we asked them some of these questions. With the help of an Hungarian translator, we interviewed them during the day about their dance traditions from the Mezőség region. In the evenings, they demonstrated these dances for us. Although they were in their 60s, 70s, and 80s, they were still spry. They danced vibrantly, smiling as they leaped and moved through each step. Two of the older men often wore Romanian Roma hats during their demonstrations and our ensuing interviews with them. These men were my inspiration to wear a black hat to the táncház at the school gymnasium. The táncház had been organized in honor of the Vişea villagers, serving as a culmination of their visit.

***

That night at the táncház, the villagers looked ready to party! They were dressed in traditional attire. The men had black slacks, plain-colored shirts, black vests, and Transylvanian hats. Each woman wore a flowy dress with a pattern on the front that resembled an apron.

My eyes were drawn to the villagers as they danced among the crowd, and they quickly became my favorite people to watch. All over the age of 60, the villagers had learned these dances as children from their friends and family, rather than in a classroom. The dance in their village had evolved much less than in more urban areas. As Csaba and I watched their movements, I realized they were doing csárdás. It was amazing to see so many people doing the steps at the same time.

I was fascinated by how each couple's movements perfectly complemented the music. The dancers held each other in a somewhat offset position. That way, the man had space on one side to do rhythmic slaps against his thighs, heels, and shoes. As the couples moved around the room in a semicircle, these slaps were used to embellish the rhythm.

I counted the basic steps. They were the same I'd learned in class: 1-and-2-and-1-2-3 and 1-and-2-and-1-2-3. Some couples maintained this basic footwork as they traveled, while others included stomps on each triple-step. The stomps indicated a change of direction. Whenever they happened, the couples began to go the opposite way in the semicircle.

Sometimes, the men and women would separate. In those moments, the men would do a solo that included slaps, stomps, and fancy steps.

"What are those slaps called?" I asked Csaba. I couldn't remember the name of all the moves, since I'd learned what they were called just a few days before during our interviews.

"They're called *ütés* or *csapás*," he replied.

"I remember!" I exclaimed. "That means 'percussion', correct?"

"Yes," Csaba said. "See how they accompany and embellish the music?"

As the men executed the ütés, the women did multiple turns around their dance partners, their dresses flaring out and accenting their spins. The men paid close attention to the women's position in order to be ready to come back together at the end of the solos. Though there was no physical contact between the dancing couple during the solos, they never lost their connection.

After a few minutes of watching, Csaba and I found dance partners and joined in.

In between the musicians' sets, there were brief lectures and demonstrations by the villagers. These were often done with live music, and ended with everyone practicing new dance steps together.

After one such demonstration, the musicians transitioned into playing a mezőségi version of korcsos. I recognized it immediately: it was what Csaba and I had practiced! The men from Vișea began to dance in front of the band, one at a time, showing their athletic prowess. We all watched and cheered.

I felt excited and nervous. I wanted to dance the choreography I'd learned with Csaba, but I felt intimidated by the large crowd watching.

I'll do it if Csaba does it with me, I thought.

I began to walk around the ballroom, looking for him. Finally, I caught sight of him. He was in the front left corner of the hall intently watching the men from Vișea dance, as if to get more inspiration from their movements.

"Csaba!" I exclaimed. "Let's go up front after these men; let's do the short routine you taught me!"

"No, I am not going," he replied.

"Why?" I asked, feeling confused. We'd worked on the choreography for weeks, and I had felt like I would be able to count on his support.

"This is your moment, Damilare," he said. "You should go. I trust that you can do it!"

I didn't like his answer! I did not feel confident enough to dance without Csaba next to me. Thus, as I watched the last of the Vișea men enter the circle to do a solo, I felt a growing sense of disappointment. I'd trained so much, but I was too afraid to take this chance. I had never done this dance by myself without Csaba dancing next to me or watching me to give corrective feedback.

When the final villager finished dancing and walked off the stage, the musicians did not stop the music. They continued to play, the space in front of them open for anyone to jump in. It was a perfect opportunity.

I stood off to the side, contemplating whether to go or not. A million thoughts ran through my head.

I'm going to be on the stage, even though I just learned this a few weeks ago... What will people think of a Black man doing Hungarian folk dance? These people have been doing these dances since they were little kids. I don't want to make a mess of it!

At the same time, I also felt excited.

This is fun! This is thrilling! This is an adventure! I can go out there and show these people how much I appreciate their culture. I can show what I have learned, and hopefully they will be pleasantly surprised.

Before I could sort through my thoughts, a rush of adrenaline propelled me to the center of the ballroom. There, in front of the musicians, I started dancing my korcsos solo. I was the center of attention.

Will they be impressed or disappointed? I wondered, focusing on each step. As I moved, my confidence built. I was remembering all the tips Csaba had given me, and it seemed like I was in time with the musicians. My nervousness began to fade, and I found myself enjoying each move of the choreography more and more.

When I finished my number and stepped off stage, I heard a roar of applause. I looked around the room and saw that everyone was smiling.

I walked back over to Csaba.

"Good job!" he said.

Then, I saw one of the Vişea villagers beckon me to come over. As I approached him, he pulled me close and patted me on the back.

"Nicely done!" he said, looking me over. "But now we have to find you a real hat!"

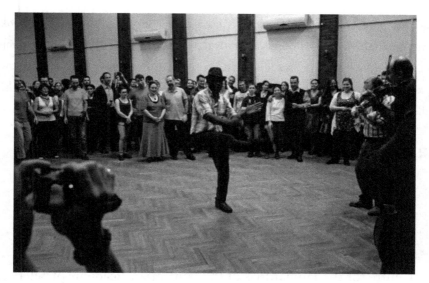

Damilare dances korcsos at the tánchéz in Szeged, Hungary
Photo credit: Department of Ethnology and Cultural Anthropology,
University of Szeged, Hungary

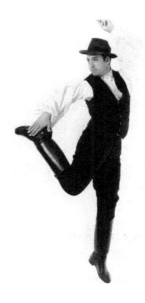

Damilare met Hungarian dancer Melles Endre (pictured above) on a Hungarian dance Facebook group while looking for photos for Dance Adventures. Melles lives in Tusnádfürdő, Hungary, and dances for a dance troupe called Háromszék Táncegyüttes in the city of Sepsiszentgyörgy. Melles took this photo of himself dancing Kalotaszegi legényes for use in this book. Damilare and Meg were impressed by his willingness to do a photoshoot for some people he had never met! This felt like a beautiful example of how dancers across the world can rise up and support one another. We are honored to feature his photo here.

Recommended resources:

Adeyeri, D. (Poster). (2016, February 9). *Damilare Adeyeri - Hungarian Folk Dance - Mezőségi Korcsos* [Video file]. Retrieved July 7, 2020, from https://www.youtube.com/watch?v=9njh0JpShko

Centre for the Humanities of the Hungarian Academy of Sciences http://db.zti.hu/neptanc_tudastar/index_en.asp

Dénes Kiss (Posterr). (2014, August 5). *Magyarpalatkai katonakísérő, de-a lungu, Romaneste-n bota és batua* [Video file]. Retrieved July 7, 2020, from https://www.youtube.com/watch?v=8IyH-8PTVyk

Elter, E. A. (Poster). (2013, June 7). *Kalamajka - Nagysajói lakodalmas (Mezőség)* [Video file]. Retrieved July 7, 2020, from https://www.youtube.com/watch?v=fwQB525v3WU

IDanceHungary. (n.d.). Retrieved July 08, 2020, from https://idancehungary.hu/

Kemecsei, Zsolt. (2017). Knowledge Base of Traditional Dances. Retrieved July 07, 2020, from http://db.zti.hu/neptanc_tudastar/index_en.asp

Kriszti60 (Poster). (2015, May 25). *Magyarszováti a Fonóban* [Video file]. Retrieved July 7, 2020, from https://www.youtube.com/watch?v=nsXrnLKocjI

Halmos, B. (n.d.). The Táncház Movement. Retrieved July 07, 2020, from http://folklife.hu/roots-to-revival/living-tradition/tanchaz-method/the-tanchaz-movement/

Martin, G. (1974). *Hungarian Folk Dances* (Vol. 7). Gyoma, Hungary: Kner Printing House.

Média Park Europe Zrt. (Producer). (2015, October 5). *Korcsos* [Video file]. Retrieved July 7, 2020, from https://www.youtube.com/watch?v=YMPVG6CObr4

Mr. Gregoriano (Poster). (2014, April 17). *Fonó zenekar - Táncházi slágerek - teljes album* [Video file]. Retrieved July 7, 2020, from https://www.youtube.com/watch?v=BX9kkWsnD7I

PSM V41 D775 Csardas Hungarian Folk Dance. (2018, January 28). Retrieved July 07, 2020, from https://commons.wikimedia.org/wiki/File:PSM_V41_D775_Csardas_hungarian_folk_dance.jpg

Szabolala (Poster). (2013, April 24). *Üsztürü - Palatkai muzsika* [Video file]. Retrieved July 7, 2020, from https://www.youtube.com/watch?v=uXuOhmh_hSU

Taylor, M. (2004). *Nineteenth and Twentieth Century Historical and Institutional Precedents of the Hungarian Dance-House Movement.* Typescript, CUNY Graduate Center, New York.

EXPLORING KIZOMBA IN ANGOLA

Carolyn McPherson

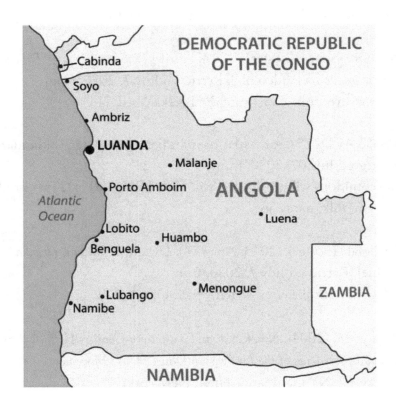

About the author: Carolyn began her dance adventures at the age of seven, when she started Scottish Highland dance classes. She has since traveled to 50 countries and danced in most of them. Highlights of her travels include dancing in front of hundreds of thousands of people in the Edinburgh Military Tattoo, as well as as well as dancing salsa in Colombia, bachata in the Dominican Republic, kizomba in Angola, and Afro-fusion in Uganda. She believes dance is a universal language and a great way to make friends all around the world. Carolyn recently resettled in her home country, Canada. She works as a yoga teacher and in her free time enjoys writing and dancing.

I spent my first Friday night in Luanda, Angola, alone in my apartment, crying.

I had travelled across the world to be here – the birthplace of kizomba – to learn more about the dance from the people who had grown up with this amazing art form. And, while I'd dreamed of visiting Angola for years, my excitement about arriving did not dissolve the obstacles between me and a great night of dancing. I didn't know where to go and I had no one to go with. Angolans had told me it was not normal to go to a club by yourself and a few expats I'd met at the airport had told me it could be dangerous to walk alone at night.

Although I had been to many African cities, Luanda was a new, somewhat mysterious destination for me. I'd met Angolans during my travels, but I'd never known anyone who had traveled to Angola. The country's strict visa policy and its incredibly high prices make it difficult to visit; therefore, the tourism industry was quite undeveloped.

Luckily enough, I'd met and befriended an Angolan government official while living abroad. He had not only helped me obtain my visa, but also found me a free place to stay: his friend's currently unused business apartment. This is how I ended up with my own furnished, air-conditioned place just blocks from the ocean.

The day before, a friendly Angolan man had helped me settle in. He was the apartment owner's driver and didn't speak any English. Before arriving, I'd used the Duolingo app to learn some Portuguese. It reminded me of the Spanish I knew, and so I quickly picked up on the language. My basics were enough for me and this man to interact effectively. He had shown me around and helped me exchange my US dollars for Angolan kwanza on the street. This, he said, was what everyone did. The rates on the street were much better than at the bank.

I felt incredibly fortunate to have this apartment. Luanda is one of the most expensive cities in the world for expats. Because oil and diamond companies subsidize expenses for their employees, apartments like this one could easily cost a few thousand dollars per month. Having a kitchen also meant I would avoid paying $80-$100 tabs at restaurants.

When the driver had left my apartment that day, he had told me to call if I needed anything. But could I call him to say I needed to go out dancing kizomba that night?

No, I thought. *That would be too much.*

I'd first discovered kizomba in 2011, while working for an NGO in Kampala, Uganda. Looking to make friends, I'd sought opportunities for partner dancing. At the social dance parties, DJs had played kizomba, bachata, merengue, and salsa music. I had learned each of these styles, and become a regular in the local dance scene. By the time I'd left the country, I was hooked. In my ensuing travels around the world, I found many places for Latin dancing. I discovered, however, that kizomba was not popular yet.

Kizomba is a partner dance that originated in Angola. The word kizomba means "party" in Kimbundu, one of the Angolan languages. During a stint teaching English in Seoul, I'd met some Angolans. They had told me about growing up with kizomba music and dancing. This is an integral part of Angolan culture, they had said, and you will see toddlers, seniors, and everyone in between moving their hips to the catchy beats. That was when the idea to visit the birthplace of kizomba had taken root in my mind. I dreamed of attending the local parties, and felt this trip would be the best way to improve my skills.

Now – three years after learning about kizomba – I was here in Angola with a 30-day tourist visa. With just four weekends to go out dancing, I knew time was precious. Sitting alone in my apartment, I felt deeply disappointed. I was missing out on an opportunity to experience the local kizomba scene. Still, the warnings I'd received felt overwhelming. Luanda was a city of great economic disparity, so armed robbery was not uncommon. The ubiquitous wealth in the country stood in stark contrast to the living conditions in the country's *musseques* (slums), and many people from poorer areas desperately wanted a piece of the pie. Crime was one way to get it.

I would later learn that most of what I'd heard was exaggerated or untrue. On that first night, however, I didn't know what to believe. I was in a foreign and unknown place, desperately wanting to go out dancing, but too afraid to leave my apartment.

When the sun came up the next day, I took action. I looked up a local yoga class and walked to the studio. As a yoga instructor, I love trying classes in every location I travel to. It's a great way to make friends and get the inside scoop on a city. After the class, I chatted with the people there, including the friendly couple who owned the studio. They told me of a place where I could dance kizomba every Sunday.

The event, I learned, was called *Kizomba na Rua* (Kizomba in the Street) and attracted some of the best dancers in the country. It was free, in an outdoor area right on the beach, and always well attended. The neighborhood was a safe place to walk alone, and all the locals who attended Kizomba na Rua were friendly. I wouldn't have any trouble finding dance partners. That sounded perfect! I felt grateful for this advice from the locals, who really knew what the conditions were like.

The next day, I went to Kizomba na Rua. Arriving early, I sat down on a bench near the plaza where the dancing would take place. I bought a homemade *mukua* (baobab) ice cream from a man walking by with a wheelbarrow-freezer contraption, and began people watching.

There on the Marginal - the name of the city's beachfront promenade - I saw both Angolans and expats jogging, walking their dogs, and taking selfies on their phones. Kids were riding bicycles and rollerblades. Young couples walked hand in hand. Behind me was the Luanda skyline, made up of high-rise office towers, luxury apartments, and old colonial structures.

Three guys wearing t-shirts that read, "Projecto Kizomba na Rua," walked up to the plaza. One of them carried a speaker, while another held extension cords. They plugged the speaker into an outlet outside a small shop selling flip-flops, connected a USB stick to the speaker, and - *voilà* - Kizomba na Rua had begun.

It was like a flash mob. As soon as the music started, people began arriving from all around. Well dressed and well coiffed, everyone seemed to be ready for a great night. Women wore nice dresses, and men wore collared shirts, pants, and shiny shoes. I walked toward the dancers with my heart pounding. This was the moment I had been waiting for! I would finally dance kizomba in Angola.

Since it was my first time there, I stood shyly off to the side. I wasn't sure of the dance etiquette here. Did people come and dance primarily with their friends, or would finding partners be easy, the way my friends at the yoga studio had predicted?

Before long, a young man approached me. He was wearing a collared shirt made with traditional Samakaka fabric, which has the same colors as the Angolan flag: yellow, red, black, and white. It is a popular fabric because wearing it shows pride in the country.

"Would you like to dance?" he asked me in Portuguese. I eagerly agreed.

My excitement about my first dance dissolved into complete presence as the young man and I began to move together. Feeling for his lead, I lost myself in the dance. When the song ended a few minutes later, I was surprised. The time had gone by too quickly. I thanked my partner and was delighted when he quickly introduced me to another lead.

From 6 p.m. to 9 p.m., I danced nonstop. The sky turned from blue to pink to orange, and finally to black. The temperature was perfect, and the surroundings beautiful. To one side of me were the ocean and palm trees. On my other side, on the top of a hill, stood an iconic old fort with a huge Angolan flag proudly flapping in the night breeze.

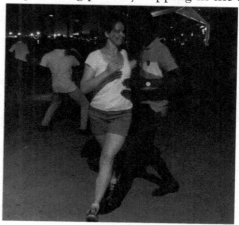

Carolyn dancing with an Angolan dancer at
Kizomba na Rua in Luanda in 2016
Photo credit: Anonymous

When Kizomba na Rua ended, I felt elated. It had been the best evening of dancing of my life. Although I had danced kizomba with people in many countries, these dances in Luanda were the best I'd ever had. The leads had challenged me with new moves, and thanks to their clear direction, I had been able to catch on quickly. Every person I met that night was a talented, patient, and considerate dance partner.

The high level of dancing was exactly what I had imagined. Angolans grow up with kizomba as a cornerstone of their culture. Kizomba music plays constantly in people's homes, at corner stores, and in the dance venues. People are constantly learning from one another. At weddings, you see grandfathers inviting their granddaughters to dance. At parties, friends show each other moves. There are studios with classes, as well, although usually only those who wish to enter a kizomba competition will enroll.

The part I enjoyed the most about dancing with the Angolans was that they smiled the entire time ~ more so than any partners I'd danced kizomba with before. Through my travels, I knew this elevated level of presence and gratitude is often common with people who have recently overcome hardship, and I imagined this could be true for many people at Kizomba na Rua. Angola's civil war had raged from 1975 to 2002, and many of the dancers that night had all known incredible strife during their lifetime. In the coming weeks, as I got to know these dancers better, they would share how challenging it had been to get by during the war.

As the organizers unplugged their speakers and packed up, people sauntered away in different directions. A few of the dancers gave me their phone numbers, saying they would take me to other events. I felt relieved. I wouldn't be sitting alone in my apartment again.

The next day, some of the dancers texted me to invite me out to another venue: Cha de Caxinde. This paid event had a very different atmosphere from Kizoma na Rua. The majority of people were in their 50s and 60s, and it was uncommon to dance with people outside your friend group. A live band played covers of old, famous kizomba songs. I danced, but also took time to sit and enjoy the fantastic music.

Over the next few weeks, I continued to explore the dance scene in Luanda. I danced with Angolans of all ages, from older men with decades of experience to incredible leads who were only eight years old. Still, out of all the events I found, Kizomba na Rua remained my favorite. Each Sunday afternoon, I would head back to the Marginal to take part. As I began to get to know people better, I received invitations to attend other interesting events.

One day, while sitting in my apartment, I got a call from a phone number I didn't recognize. Picking up, I was greeted by a friendly voice.

"Hello Carolyn, this is Adilson," a man said in Portuguese. "We've danced several times at Kizomba na Rua, and I got your phone number from a friend."

I didn't recognize Adilson's voice or his name, but I was curious to know why he was calling.

"I'm a performer," he explained. "I often dance on national television, and there is an afternoon entertainment segment that wants to highlight how kizomba is danced abroad. They'd like me to perform with a foreigner, and then we will discuss how kizomba is evolving worldwide."

This sounded like a great opportunity, and I agreed to attend. Adilson said he would pick me up the next day. Without any direction on what to wear, I had decided on black pants, a black top, a white blazer, and high-heeled dance shoes.

As I exited my apartment building, I was surprised to see a white van waiting with a colorful "TV Zimbo" logo on the side

The back door slid open, and I saw familiar faces. I immediately recognized Adilson, as well as a few other people from Kizomba na Rua. We would all be dancing together, Adilson explained.

As we drove out of downtown Luanda, the houses got smaller and smaller. We passed many convenience stores, gas stations, hair and nail shops, and trucks selling hamburgers. There were men gathered on the street at every red light displaying the wares they had to sell: carpets, cockroach killers, maps of Angola, and jeans. After about 20 minutes, we arrived at a gated complex that contained the headquarters for TV

Zimbo.

A few people from the television station ushered us into a waiting room, where they touched up our makeup and told us to wait until we were called. Everything was filmed live, so they needed to carefully coordinate each act.

Half an hour later, when the show cut to a commercial break, they called us to the set. The two television hosts, a man and a woman, were waiting for us. Both were fantastically gorgeous. The man was lean and muscular, with a bright white smile. He wore nice pants and a white, button-down shirt rolled up past his wrists. The woman was tall and had her black hair twisted up into a messy bun. She wore a fitted black dress and black heels.

They gave instructions on where to dance and what our cues would be, and they chatted with us politely.

"You really came to Angola just to dance kizomba?" the woman asked me, clearly surprised.

"Yes," I said. "It's been a wonderful experience so far."

Our conversation was cut short as the cameraman counted us in.

"We're live in 5, 4, 3, 2..."

The hosts didn't miss a beat. They smiled broadly as the show began, and introduced us.

"Today we have guests from the kizomba performance team "Fenomeno Do Semba" here, as well as Carolyn McPherson, who is visiting from Canada. After a demonstration, we will talk about kizomba, and about how people dance kizomba abroad."

A traditional Angolan kizomba song began to play, and Adilson invited me to dance. After about a minute, the hosts cut in. The male host asked me to dance, while the female host danced with Adilson. The host was surprised at how well I could follow his lead.

When the song ended, we sat down on couches in front of the television camera, and began to talk about the growing popularity of kizomba around the world.

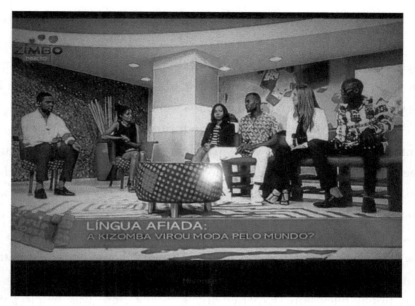

Carolyn's interview on TV Zimbo in 2016 about the differences between kizomba in Angola and abroad. Pictured are the hosts, Carolyn (in the white blazer), and other invited guests.
Photo credit: Carolyn McPherson

While many cities around the world have a kizomba social dance scene, most people outside of Angola do not know how kizomba is traditionally danced. In Angola, most dance venues play songs with Portuguese lyrics. Couples focus on continuous movement to the music, staying grounded with soft knees, and having close, chest-to-chest connection. Perhaps the most important ingredient of kizomba, however, is the *ginga*.

While the simple definition of ginga is how a dancer moves their hips, the meaning is deeper than that. Ginga in Angolan kizomba is about rhythm, creativity, and style. It is unique to each dancer, and, because Angolans are so steeped in kizomba, they each have a refined way of moving.

As kizomba gained popularity worldwide, it evolved from its traditional form and fused with other styles. Now, when people abroad say they are dancing kizomba, odds are they are doing urban kiz. The "kiz" in the name indicates that this dance was influenced by kizomba.

In urban kiz, people most often dance to instrumental music or songs sung in French or English. Dancers will pause, do contra tempo moves in accordance with the music, or add in styling from hip hop or other modern styles of dance. They also sometimes include acrobatics.

"There are different opinions about this style," the television host pointed out. "While many Angolans are proud that a part of our culture is becoming so popular, others do not like how the dance is being modified or how many people calling themselves kizomba teachers are actually teaching urban kiz."

As the segment wrapped up, I realized again how fortunate I was to have the chance to dance kizomba in Angola. I was grateful for the people that I met, like Adilson, and for the cool opportunity to appear on national television. Experiencing kizomba here was helping me appreciate the dance on a much deeper level.

Not long after my television debut, I realized my visa was about to expire. But I wasn't ready to leave. So I gathered the necessary paperwork, paid a fee, and submitted a visa extension through the Ministry of External Relations. Within a few days, I had been granted another three months in Angola.

As it turned out, my first 30 days were just the beginning of an incredible adventure. By the end of my four-month stay, I had improved my Portuguese by speaking with my new friends, taken private dance lessons with Adilson and other amazing Angolan teachers, deepened my passion for kizomba music, and improved my ginga. Now, when I dance abroad or in my home country of Canada, people often say, "There's something different about your dancing! Where did you learn?"

When it was time to leave Angola, I was crying again. So much had changed since that first night when I was alone in my apartment. I was sad to leave my new friends and this country that had warmly welcomed me. As my plane took off, I looked down at the beach, the islands, the skyscrapers, the musseques, and the baobab trees. I knew I would be back, and I knew I would never waste another night in Luanda.

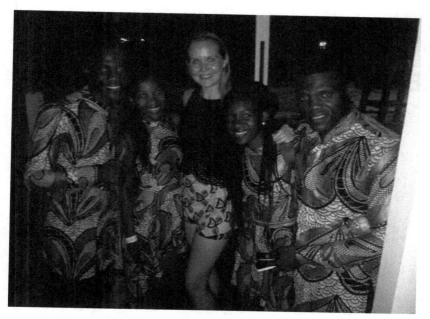

Members of the Angolan dance group Fenomeno do Semba and Carolyn in 2016. From left to right: Adilson, Thelma, Carolyn, Nelinha, and Jone.
Photo credit: Anonymous

Recommended resources:

Dancing Semba / Kizomba on the Street in Angola: Adilson Maíza and Carolyn McPherson [Video file]. (2017, October 14). Retrieved July 7, 2020, from https://www.youtube.com/watch?v=dNfX8HI90JE

Moorman, M. J. (2008). *Intonations: A Social History of Music and Nation in Luanda, Angola, from 1945 to Recent Times.* Athens, OH: Ohio University Press.

LESSONS IN DANCE EDUCATION

Gabrielle Brigida Macalintal

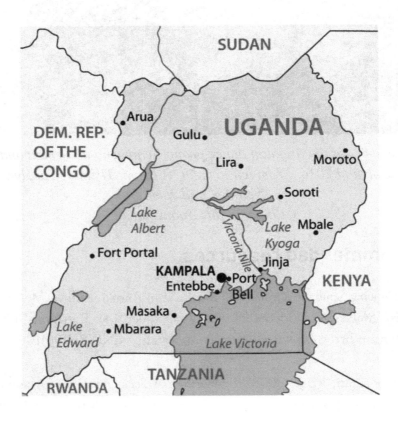

About the author: Gabrielle Brigida Macalintal is a New York State-certified dance educator who lives in White Plains, NY. She has taught all grade levels and demographics in public schools over the past decade, with a focus on middle school. Gabrielle is passionate about bringing dance education to young people who may not otherwise have the opportunity to participate. She focuses both on cultivating her students' artistic expression and on their general development into empowered young adults. Most recently, she presented her middle school curriculum model for multicultural dance education at the National Dance Education Organization's annual conference in San Diego (2018), and contributed to the New York City Department of Education's Arts and Special Projects Compendium on Teaching Students with Disabilities in the Arts (2017). She received her BA in dance and arts in education from Hobart and William Smith Colleges, and an MA in dance education from NYU Steinhardt.

When I was 17 years old, I met with a guidance counselor to talk about my college career. He was an older, bald man in his mid-60s who wore a cardigan and thin, wire-rimmed glasses. And, while he had years of experience, I was about to throw him a curveball.

"What do you want to major in?" he asked me, smiling kindly.

"Psychology and dance," I responded, sitting up straight. "I love learning about the mind, and I love to move."

He blinked and shifted slightly, his smile fading to a frown.

"My daughter majored in psychology and ended up a bartender."

I found myself feeling slightly annoyed and wishing he were more supportive. He hadn't even bothered to mention dance, which I assume seemed even more ridiculous in his mind.

"You need to make sure your major has a career path," he said. "Otherwise you'll end up like she did."

I left the guidance counselor's office feeling frustrated, but not dissuaded. When I was growing up in a small town in upstate New York, few people in my community understood that dance could be a career. Most had never met someone who was gainfully employed as a performer or full-time dance teacher. Still, I knew this was my path: at a young age, I'd realized dance was more to me than just an art form.

To say that I lived to dance is not an understatement. I looked forward to my annual dance studio recitals more than Christmas. As a shy kid, I felt overlooked and misunderstood in many environments. In my dance classes, however, I felt seen and appreciated. On stage, I was in my element: confident, expressive, and fully present in the moment.

I saw dance as a beacon of inspiration and possibility. It connected me to the highest version of myself, and it gave me a voice. Over the next few years, as I studied psychology and dance in college (despite the guidance counselor's misgivings), I realized my mission: to become an advocate for the arts who helped students find their confidence, self-expression, and voice through dance, just as I had.

This led to my decision to pursue a master's in dance education at New York University Steinhardt. As I prepared to enter NYU in the fall of 2010, I could never have guessed how much I would learn, much less that some of my most eye-opening moments would happen during a study abroad program in Uganda. At that time, all I knew was that I wanted to develop the skills necessary to engage even the shyest, most reluctant, or most nervous students. I wanted to be an ambassador for dance who connected students to this living, breathing art form.

In my first days on campus at NYU, I battled imposter syndrome. Surrounded by seasoned dancers and dance educators, I worried about being good enough. I wondered if my dance training in upstate New York had been adequate, and felt embarrassed that I didn't have as much teaching experience as many of my peers.

No one else seemed worried about my qualifications. In fact, everyone at Steinhardt was very welcoming. This included Deborah Damast, the artistic director of the Kaleidoscope Dance Company. Deborah taught one of my elective classes, and I liked her from the start. A short, spunky blonde, she was a kind and dynamic teacher. I also looked up to her for the role she played in the world of dance education. Deborah took part in state- and national-level dance organizations, ran various programs in the dance department, and led Kaleidocope's arts inreach program.

In class the first day, Deborah explained how our year together would unfold.

"For the next few months, I'll teach you the Kaleidoscope dance-making model," she said. "We use this model to give students the tools they need to take ownership of their learning. Rather than telling them what to do, we would teach them the history and cultural context of a dance, as well as the movement vocabulary. Afterward, students would turn the movements into their own choreography."

I took copious notes, as I knew I would be teaching classes using the Kaleidoscope model in the spring. This was a much different instruction style than I had learned growing up, and one that aligned with my teaching goals. Previously, when I had taken classes or taught, I'd followed a designated curriculum. Never had I seen a flexible model that pulled forth each individual's creativity.

"Let's jump in," Deborah said excitedly, motioning us to follow her to a whiteboard in the corner of the room, where she had hung a map of Uganda. "For the next few weeks, I'll use the Kaleidoscope model to teach you a traditional Ugandan dance called *Kimwanda*."

Deborah pointed to a southwestern region of the country.

"Kimwanda is danced by men and women from the Bahiru tribe of the Bankankole people who live here," she said. "The dance is done to worship the gods and request help in times of crisis."

There are hundreds of different dances across Uganda, Deborah went on to explain. They come from the country's 56 different tribes, which span Uganda's four kingdoms. Dances in Uganda and across the African continent bear a testament to the meaning of *vernacular dance*, or "dance of the people." The dances were all created for different reasons, from celebrating nature to honoring life events such as birth, marriage, and death.

"In Uganda, there are many different languages, as well," Deborah told us. "Many people speak English, however, since Uganda was colonized by England until 1962."

As Deborah spoke, she passed around a few items. There was a common instrument in Ugandan music – an *engoma* drum – and children's books that contained illustrations and photographs of traditional Ugandan dances. When the books came to me, I took my time flipping through the pages.

I have a lot to learn, I thought. Ugandan dance, as well as the idea of incorporating history, geography, and music appreciation into my classes, was new to me. Furthermore, having grown up in a white suburban family, I hadn't learned much about African culture until now.

Over the next few weeks, Deborah taught us the moves of Kimwanda in a call-and-response fashion. She didn't give us counts. Instead, she danced, and we followed along. This was very different from how I'd learned modern and ballet. Deborah's classes didn't focus on lines, technique, and precision. They focused on expression, energy, and individual style.

"This dance is not about being too careful or moving in a certain way!" Deborah would tell us again and again. "You will all look slightly different, and that's just fine!"

One day, at the end of class, Deborah called us over to make an announcement.

"For the past six years, I've taken a group of NYU graduate students to Uganda for a dance-focused exchange," she said. "This program was started by Sylvia Nagginda Luswata, who is the queen of the Buganda Kingdom, which includes Uganda's capital city of Kampala. The program is a partnership between NYU and Makerere University there."

The exchange was designed to help students become better dance teachers, Deborah went on. While in Uganda, participants would work alongside Makerere students, using the Kaleidoscope dance-making model to teach classes to local youth and adults. They would also take classes in Ugandan dance from Makerere professors. Participants would be given the chance to be on both sides – to be the student and the instructor – in order to best reflect on their own pedagogy. The experience would culminate in a joint performance with all participants.

I'm going, I thought. There was no hesitation. In my gut, I knew this was the next step in my education. My classes with Deborah were already challenging my ideas about dance instruction. Clearly, there was more to explore about what it meant to be the best teacher possible. I could only imagine how much I would learn studying in Uganda.

"What do I need to do to be ready?" I asked Deborah that day.

"Enroll in the course called 'Intercultural Dance,'" she replied. "It's taught by Alfdaniels Mabingo, who is from Uganda. He's a wealth of information."

The next semester, I joined 20 of my fellow graduate students in Mabingo's class. We were all sitting on the floor of the dance studio chatting and stretching when Mabingo entered the room on the first day.

"It's great to have you all here," he said, beaming. "My name is Alfdaniels Mabingo, and I know many of you are going to Uganda next year. You will love it!"

Mabingo explained that he had graduated from Makerere University before becoming a professor there. He had met Deborah while studying under Jill Pribyl at Makerere and taking part in the first study abroad course with NYU in 2007. Now, he was here researching intercultural dance as a Fulbright Scholar. More specifically, he wanted to know how to best teach Eastern styles of dance in the West.

"There isn't much East African dance being taught and performed in the United States," he explained, "so it's a very exciting area of research. I also love sharing more about arts education in Uganda with aspiring dance teachers like you. Most people are surprised to hear how high a priority the arts are in my country."

In Uganda, Mabingo said, dance is woven into the culture and is a facet of identity, tradition, pride, worship, celebration, and rites of passage. It is so important that schools teach dance and music with the same rigor with which they teach history and math. Furthermore, the approach was holistic, much closer to the Kaleidoscope model I'd learned than any dance class I'd taken before my experience at NYU.

"When I teach you a dance, I'll share its historical and cultural context, as well as the songs, rituals, or stories that go along with it," Mabingo said.

Is there really a whole country where this holistic approach to dance education is the norm? I marveled. While I knew this sort of arts education existed in the United States, it was rare. In most places, dance is still considered an extracurricular activity.

Over the next few months, Mabingo taught us about dances known by most Ugandans, as well as those done by specific tribal groups. Of the latter, the Imbalu circumcision ceremony most fascinated me.

This ceremony is only performed by Uganda's Bagisu people in Eastern Uganda and is centuries old. When young men come of age, their village hosts an event that includes each young man's circumcision, as well as specific songs, dances, and other rituals.

Mabingo said the origin story of this ritual tells of a man who was known for stealing other men's wives. The council of elders summoned the man and prescribed circumcision as a punishment. The circumcision did not stop his philandering, however. In fact, it did quite the opposite: women found the man even more alluring. When the local men discovered this, they circumcised themselves in order to compete.

The more I learned about the breadth and diversity of Uganda's dance traditions, the more excited I became about my upcoming visit.

***

One year later, as my NYU colleagues and I boarded our flight to East Africa, I set an intention: I would soak up every moment, learning as much as possible in order to be a better teacher and advocate for the arts.

After twenty-four hours and two layovers, I arrived at Entebbe International Airport and emerged from the plane into pressing darkness. Uganda, I would soon learn, could not afford much of the infrastructure I was used to in the United State, including street lights. And, although I would later get used to this, it was unnerving at first. I was in a new place and could not take stock of my surroundings.

After collecting our luggage, we headed through customs, where several Ugandan students from Makerere University were waiting for us. They greeted us enthusiastically and helped us load our luggage onto a large bus. With this warm welcome, I felt some of my nervousness dissipate. I was grateful to be having this experience with my NYU cohort and eager to know our Ugandan counterparts better.

As we drove into the night, I saw little but darkness. The long road was lined by deep ditches and telephone poles with loose wires. There were few people, but occasionally a stray goat or dog would wander across the road. Everyone on the bus was quiet, but I sensed a heightened alertness. While we were tired from traveling, we were also taking in this new place that was different than what we knew in the United States. I wondered how long it would take each of us to adjust to this new environment.

We soon arrived at the Fang Fang Hotel, which had gotten its name from the Chinese immigrants who owned the establishment. The China–Uganda connection would be evident throughout our stay. The two countries have a close relationship, as China was one of the first nations to recognize Uganda's independence. Many businesses in Uganda are owned by Chinese people, and you see billboards in Mandarin along the roads.

My room at the Fang Fang was clean and basic. That night, I climbed under the mosquito net that covered the four-poster bed and quickly fell asleep to the hum of the electric fan.

After a simple breakfast of fruit, eggs, and ginger tea the next morning, we began our studies with the students and faculty from the Makerere University Music, Dance, and Drama Department. We met in the gymnasium of a local primary school: a large space with floor-to-ceiling windows on each side. These windows provided ample light for us, as well as prime viewing for many curious, young Ugandan children.

Our rigorous daily schedule included lectures, in addition to instruction in different traditional songs and dances that dated back to the beginning of the Buganda Kingdom, where the city of Kampala is located today. Our teachers emphasized that learning Bugandan dances allowed us to experience where we were working and living in a deeper way. We learned about traditions from the other regions, too. This is how we came to understand more about Uganda's various clans, royal history, and cultural diversity.

My favorite of the dances we learned was the mushroom dance, called *amaggunju*. Amaggunju was originally created for the boy king, Mulondo. He was crowned while still an infant after his father died during a hunt. Since women were not allowed to ascend to the throne, Mulondo "ruled" through his mother, who always sat nearby.

Mulondo's mother was from the Mushroom Clan, and she depended on her brothers to help keep the baby both entertained and protected. The moves they used later evolved into the dynamic amaggungu dance.

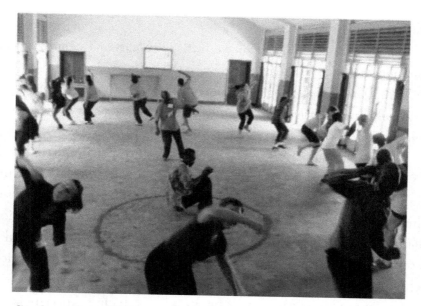

*Students from NYU and Makerere University, led by Herbert
Mukungu, dancing in the gymnasium of Nakasero Primary School
Photo credit: Rebecca Hoffman*

Originally only performed by Baganda men from the Mushroom Clan, the dance is now done by men and women of any ethnicity or clan affiliation. All the dancers wear *raffia* skirts and goat skins that make amaggunju's characteristic high jumps and kicks easier to execute, and women tie long strips of goat hide around their waist to exaggerate the movement of their hips. Ankle rattles accentuate rhythms tapped out by dancers' feet.

"Bend your knees more, and imagine you're pulling the mushrooms from the ground!" the Ugandan students reminded us as we practiced the moves. "Remember, that move shows the harvest of the mushrooms!"

What amazed me further about these songs, dances, and stories was that so many people knew them. Singing and dancing thus connected everyone, and was a way to engage with the community and honor the past. That week, I took copious notes in my journal, not just about my experience, but about how I could apply the lessons to engage students in my future classes.

Dance class is about more than cultivating flexibility and stamina. It's an opportunity to nurture creativity and connection.

Taking part in something universal is a powerful experience of unity.

A holistic approach makes dancing accessible to students with different learning styles.

This style of dancing and learning was so fun that I poured myself into the experience, putting more energy into my first week of dancing in Uganda than into any previous performance project. To my surprise, rather than feeling exhausted by it, I found the dance immersion magnified my energy and increased my wellbeing. Not only did I thoroughly enjoy each day, but I found myself waking up earlier, sleeping better at night, and even experiencing improved digestion.

The experience was nurturing in ways I hadn't known dance education could be. I felt no sense of competition with my peers; only connection. I felt inspired and creative, without the pressure to get moves exactly right. Our Ugandan teachers talked about rhythm in a way that created a sense of togetherness and took away my fear of messing something up. They said rhythm is an inherent part of our humanity.

"There is no correct way to move," they told us. "All you need to do is listen to the music. Whatever dance you create is a perfect expression of your unique voice."

One night, after a day of dancing, I climbed into bed with my journal at the Fang Fang hotel. To a soundtrack of crickets and the hum of the electric fan, I began to write.

These classes promote inclusiveness, connection, and creativity. They have the power to help students become as comfortable with their imagination as they are with technology. If I want to help students recover a sense of personal and community identity, and to learn to trust themselves rather than look for a "right" answer, I must apply what I'm learning here in Uganda.

The next week, Deborah and Jill Pribyl, former Fulbright Scholar and now a professor of dance at Makerere University's Department of Performing Arts and Film, prepared us to teach the Ugandan children.

They began by breaking our group into trios. I was paired with Herman Bagonza from Makerere and Corrine Colon from NYU. Bagonza had stood out to me from the first day. He had an infectious, warm spirit, and was always humming a song or rhythm. Corrine, a dancer from Florida with a background in cheer and jazz dance, brought her experience as a member of her college dance team and a dance studio instructor. Her presence would infuse our planning with a sense of discipline and rigor.

Corrine, Bagonza, and I were assigned to students aged 11–18. We would teach them moves from our genres of expertise, and then encourage them to create their own choreographies for the upcoming performance at the National Theatre in Kampala. We would have just one week to make sure they were ready.

"These kids come from a variety of backgrounds," Jill explained. "Some are from orphanages and children's centers, and may have been through traumatic events such as the loss of their parents. Other children are from upper-middle-class families who can afford tuition at the Queen's National Ballet School."

While some of the students would be instantly open and trusting, others might initially feel uncomfortable, she told us. Many would have trouble making eye contact or would be afraid to speak up.

As Jill spoke, Deborah nodded along.

"Remember, too, that the children who have ballet training are not necessarily the best dancers when it comes to the traditional dances," Deborah said. "The young people from children's centers perform traditional dances and are experts. Many learned these dances when they were little and the rhythms, songs, and movements are a part of their lived experience."

Deborah added that compassion needed to be central to our teaching.

"Lead with care, and speak clearly and slowly," she said. "Remember that students have varying levels of English. Stay positive and encourage them to ask questions. This way, they can practice their language skills and grow their confidence."

I felt a wave of compassion move through my body. While I had not experienced traumatic events as a child, I knew what it was like to worry about fitting in, to have an adult talk down to you, or to feel that others doubted your abilities. I felt protective over these young people. I wanted to give them the best experience possible and to make sure they knew they each had an important role to play.

"The energy you bring will be important," Jill said. "You can be playful and fun, but don't forget to maintain a structured learning environment. Both of these are critical if you want students to feel safe trying new things."

Finally, Deborah and Jill emphasized that we needed to pay careful attention to group dynamics. To encourage new friendships and help the children build confidence, we were to create groups that mixed students from different backgrounds.

A few days later, upon arriving at Queen's National Ballet School, Bagonza, Corrine, and I headed to a downstairs space to meet our students. Our assigned studio was lovely. It included a bright, airy room with auditorium-style seating, tall windows, and a patio outside the door from which you could look out at the manicured gardens. As we entered, we saw that the students were already hanging out in separate groups, just as we'd been told they would.

As the clock ticked closer to the start of class, I felt a nervous flutter in my stomach move up into my chest. This was the first time I would teach dance in a culture different from my own. Furthemore, it was time to test what we'd learned at NYU and here in Uganda. This felt deeply vulnerable. We wouldn't be using someone else's curriculum. We'd created these classes on our own, which meant we would fully own the outcome of our work—the successes and the shortcomings.

Reminding myself that Corinne and Bagonza had my back, I took some deep breaths and tried to relax. Soon, the energy shifted into excitement. We had spent the last few weeks preparing, and I felt confident that we were ready.

"Let's get started!" I said to Corrine and Bagonza. Bagonza began setting up the music, and Corinne and I walked over to gather the students. As we approached them, several girls bounded up to us.

"What are we going to be learning?" they asked us.

"Jazz and hip hop," I answered.

"Oh!" they said. "We love hip hop! We just saw some in Chris Brown's new music video!" Without any prompting, they began showing us moves involving sharp twists at the hips. I loved their confidence and felt intrigued that a Chris Brown video that had been popular in the United States five years ago, was now having its heyday in Uganda. I'd never considered that songs might become popular around the world at different times.

"That looks pretty good!" I said to the girls, encouraging them. "I think you'll do just fine. Head on in! We're about to get started!"

I smiled to myself as the girls lined up across the front of the room. This mirrored the dynamic I knew back in the United States, where the outgoing children often came forward first.

A group of young boys from one of the children's centers hung back. They were clearly shy and self-conscious, but trying to appear cool and nonchalant about being in a dance class. They had hard expressions, but I wasn't going to be fooled.

"Come on!" I called warmly. "This is going to be fun! We're doing hip hop!"

Hearing this, one of the boys lit up. He began translating what I'd said from English to Luganda for his friends.

"Oh!" I heard them say. "Hip hop! Chris Brown!"

As they made their way onto the dance floor, Bagonza began a call-and-response clapping and vocal drill to draw the students into a circle. As the students copied Bagonza, the energy in the room shifted. I felt a greater sense of ease and connection, as we all began to share the same rhythm. I imagined the students felt the energy change, too. They began to smile, and their bodies seemed to relax. The class was starting off strong; this was our first opportunity to make sure everyone felt included and ready to proceed with the day's workshop. Our efforts seemed to be working.

Bagonza continued to lead, and his instruction felt like a

spontaneous game of follow-the-leader. While he had been happy to lesson plan with us before class, he was obviously also comfortable with adjusting that plan as he went. He moved fluidly through a warmup, and then taught some movements from a traditional Ugandan dance. Whenever he was about to teach something new, he transitioned with a quick story or a call-and-response song. It grabbed the students' attention.

Corinne and I taught next, using the Kaleidoscope model. Corinne introduced a jazzy, cheer-style combination that included staccato, angular motions. I then gave the students material to work with, pulling from my experience on my college's hip hop and step team. I conjured up a small body rhythm combination that used claps, stomping, and slaps against the side of the thigh as percussion.

The students picked up all our choreography quickly. We then divided them into groups, making sure that they had the opportunity to work with other students they didn't know. By the end of class that day, each group had created new ways to combine and style the moves. The students were experimenting with partnering, timing, and adding in new variations and ideas of their own. They were laughing together and working as a team. Even the young men who had been so reluctant to join class at the beginning were engaged with their group members.

This felt like a success not just for the students, but also for us as teachers. Deborah and Jill had told us that, as dance educators, we must not just focus on technical and artistic achievement. Rather, our goal in Uganda and everywhere else was to foster engagement, self-expression, and artistic collaboration—especially in a group of children whose members had experienced trauma, hardship, and language and cultural barriers, and who hardly knew us or each other at all.

Although this had been a collaborative effort, as class wrapped up that day, I also felt a strong sense of personal accomplishment. My contribution had mattered, both to my fellow teachers and to the students.

In the coming days, the students became more and more comfortable with us and one another. We joked more and shared more about our life experience. The children were exceptionally curious. They wanted to know where we were from, all about our families, and whether we personally knew celebrities such as Obama and (of course) Chris Brown. I'd never developed this level of relationship and comfort with a group of students so quickly.

All the while, we continued to teach dance. With every lesson, I felt like I was transitioning from a guest in the country to a key facilitator in a dance exchange experience. My ability to lead and teach had clearly improved since I'd arrived at NYU nearly a year and a half earlier.

After a week, it was time for our final performance at the National Theater in Kampala. Each year, this performance sells out. It is well advertised throughout the capital city, and people look forward to attending this annual collaborative extravaganza of music, dancing, and singing by artists from Makerere and NYU.

By the time we were scheduled to go on, a cacophony of voices echoed through the auditorium. As the emcee hushed the crowd, we huddled backstage with the students. We gave each other a squeeze around the shoulders, and Corinne, Bagonza, and I whispered, "Good luck," to the students. They would be going first, and they were ready! As the lights over the audience dimmed and the stage lights came on, our students made their entrance.

Wearing brightly colored "I Love NYC" t-shirts, they moved across the stage like a flock of beautiful, graceful birds. They carried themselves with certainty and courage, and they radiated joy as they moved through their choreography. We had taught them moves, but they had made this dance their own. Seeing their happiness, I felt my own soul take flight. The experience confirmed that I was gaining the skills required to empower young people of many different backgrounds through dance.

We were only able to watch for a few minutes before we had to go get ready for our own performance. We'd prepared a mashup of traditional Ugandan dances, including kimwanda and amaggunju, for this special night. The crowd loved seeing our NYU cohort perform alongside our Makerere counterparts. As we danced, our students cheered wildly from the sides of the stage.

The performance that night stretched for more than two hours with a variety of incredible duets and smaller group pieces in between the larger acts. We also had a dance battle between the kids and the grownups to the music of – you guessed it – Chris Brown. The evening was topped off by a women's dance to "We Run the World" by Beyoncé. By the time I heard the last notes in the music, the sense of family between everyone on stage was palpable. I felt deeply connected to, and accepted by, my NYU cohort, my students, and my new friends at Makerere.

As I boarded the plane home, I took stock of all I'd learned. I promised myself that I would continue to use an intentional, integrative teaching style that incorporated history, music, and cultural lessons into my dance classes. Furthermore, I would always do my best to lead with compassion and enthusiasm, as well as to emphasize the inherent value of creativity and learning.

I also saw the opportunity to expand my range as a teacher. After taking my seat, I jotted down notes about the organic, spontaneous instruction style that Bagonza had expertly modeled. I wanted to play with embodying more of that energy in my instruction.

Moving forward, whenever I taught a new class or found myself in a new environment, I would remember my first day teaching the Ugandan students. I would remind myself of my training, focus on my goal to empower students to dance, and breathe until my uncertainty transitioned into excitement.

Today, I know I've made good on my promise to myself. As I write this story, eight years after receiving my master's, I realize the lessons from my graduate school years are so ingrained in me that I rarely even think about them. Wisdom from Deborah, Mabingo, Jill, Bagonza, and everyone else I met during my time at NYU and abroad in Uganda has allowed me to become a teacher who can, and does, make an impact.

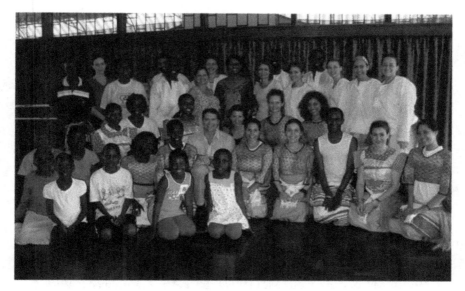

Students and faculty from NYU and Makerere University take a group shot with Sylvia Nagginda Luswata (center), Queen of the Buganda Kingdom, which is one of the four kingdoms in Uganda
Photo credit: Rebecca Hoffman

Recommended resources:

Asiimwe, A., & Ibanda, G. F. (2008). *Dances of Uganda*. Kampala, Uganda: Tourguide Publications.

Blanc, J. (2020, March 03). Cultural Mistakes to Avoid in Uganda. Retrieved July 08, 2020, from https://kabiza.com/kabiza-wilderness-safaris/cultural-mistakes-to-avoid-in-uganda/

Blanc, J. (2020, January 06). Uglish – Ugandan English – 101 for Visitors to Uganda. Retrieved July 08, 2020, from https://kabiza.com/kabiza-wilderness-safaris/uglish-ugandan-english-101-for-visitors-to-uganda/

Blanc, J. (2017, July 08). What to Wear in Kampala - Entebbe - Uganda. Retrieved July 08, 2020, from https://kabiza.com/kabiza-wilderness-safaris/what-to-wear-in-kampala-uganda/

Byakutaaga, S. C. (2006). *Tips on Ugandan Cultures*. Kampala, Uganda: Tourguide Publications.

Eichstaedt H. (2013). *First Kill Your Family: Child Soldiers of Uganda and the Lord's Resistance Army*. Chicago, IL: Lawrence Hill Books.

Elderkin N. (Director). (2010). *Bouncing Cats* [Motion picture]. USA: Red Bull Media House.

Fine, S., & Fine, A. N. (Directors). (2007). *War/Dance* [Motion picture]. USA: THINKFilm.

Hodd, M., & Carswell, M. (1997). *East Africa Handbook: With Kenya, Tanzania, Uganda and Ethiopia*. Bath, UK: Footprint Handbooks.

Kofago Dance Ensemble (Producer). (2017, May 9). *Uganda 2017 NYU* [Video file]. Retrieved July 7, 2020, from https://vimeo.com/216716700/0c8904665a

Macdonald K. (Director). (2006). *The Last King of Scotland* [Motion picture]. United Kingdom and Germany: Fox Searchlight Pictures.

Nair, M. (Director). (2016). *Queen of Katwe* [Video file]. USA: Walt Disney Studios Motion Pictures.

Natabaalo, G., & Hitchen, J. (2018, January 16). 24 Things to Know Before You Go to Kampala. Retrieved July 08, 2020, from https://roadsandkingdoms.com/2017/24-things-to-know-before-you-go-to-kampala/

Sweikar, M. (2007). *Mzungu: A Notre Dame Student in Uganda*. Nashville, TN: Cold Tree Press.

A LINDY HOP LOVE STORY

Tina Shield

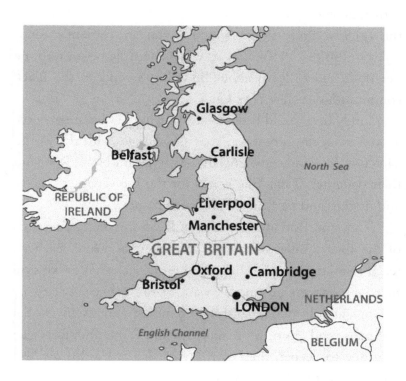

About the author: Tina began dancing lindy hop in Seattle, Washington, USA, in 2oO2. After learning the basic steps on the social dance floor, she began traveling to attend workshops with renowned teachers, including Frankie Manning, one of the original lindy hoppers and a star in Harlem's Savoy Ballroom in the 1930s. This is when she truly began to hone her skills and to learn about lindy hop's roots in the Black communities of New York City.

Lindy hop would become one of Tina's greatest passions, as well as an important way that she engages with the world. Tina now lives in Leeds, England, with her husband, Rob, and their daughter, Talia. She works for the University of Leeds, and teaches and performs with Swing Dance Leeds.

Tina and Rob are working on becoming better stewards of the Black American dances that they, as white teachers, teach to a largely white, European audience. They make sure that new dancers are made aware of the dance's origins by talking about dance history, handing out educational materials, and posting on social media. Tina and Rob also continue to deepen their own knowledge of the history and social context of these dances.

Tina holds a BA in theatre from Concordia College and an MA in theatre and global development from the University of Leeds.

In the autumn of 2009, I arrived in Leeds, England, ready to begin my master's in theatre and global development at the University of Leeds.

I'd secured funding for my schooling via a Rotary Ambassadorial Scholarship, which required that I not just pursue my degree, but also promote cultural exchange between my home country and my host country through talks at local Rotary Clubs. There was one aspect of American culture that I was very keen to share about – lindy hop – so I included information about this American-born dance in all my presentations.

Lindy hop, the original swing dance, was born in the Black communities of Harlem in New York City. Hearing the foot-tapping jazz played by big bands led by musicians such as Duke Ellington and Benny Goodman, members of the Black community were inspired to dance. The dances they created, including lindy hop, became wildly popular in the local ballrooms.

In the 50s, as music such as rock and roll became more popular, the era of big band swing and lindy hop came to an end. In the 1980s, however, the dance experienced a revival when dancers in New York City, California, Stockholm, and the United Kingdom each independently searched for original lindy hop dancers in order to learn the dance from them. At this time, the original dancers – Al Minns, Pepsi Bethel, Frankie Manning, and Norma Miller – came out of retirement and began to tour the world teaching lindy hop.

The first time I saw lindy hop was in 2002, when a friend invited me out to a social dance. I'd taken a few ballroom swing lessons in college, but what I saw when I arrived was very different. While some people were doing the basic steps I'd learned, others by the DJ booth were doing something very different. It was more athletic, and infinitely more interesting. They were dancing lindy hop, my friend told me, and I was immediately hooked. I started going to weekend workshops and social dancing four nights a week.

Everyone at the dances was friendly and encouraging, even though I didn't know what I was doing. Practicing, learning, and developing as a dancer was so much fun that it didn't feel like work, and the reward was incredible: I was able to have better and better dances with my partners on the social floor. After a few months of this informal lindy hop immersion, I signed up for my first camp: a whole week of dancing with teachers from all over the world, including the legendary Frankie Manning, one of the best lindy hoppers from the 1930s, who was still sharing his love of the dance at nearly 90 years old.

After those first couple of years in Seattle, life took me to a few different places. Wherever I could find lindy hoppers, however, I knew I'd have a ready-made group of friends. With thriving lindy hop scenes not just across the United States, but all over the world, it was often easy to make connections.

Through Rotary, I had lined up a place to live before I left the United States. Fresh off the flight to London and the three-hour train journey north to Leeds, I arrived at my new home. I'd be staying in a back-to-back terraced house, a common style of home built during the Industrial Revolution that was still very prevalent in this area of England.

My landlord, who fully embraced the history of the place, had even installed a traditional laundry dryer that hung from the ceiling in the kitchen over the old fireplace. I could move it up and down on a pulley to load and unload the clothes. The idea of having a washing machine in the kitchen and hanging clothes around the house to dry was one of the many things I would need to get used to in this country that was so similar to, and yet so different from, my own.

As I prepared to start classes, fifteen years after receiving my bachelor's from a tiny liberal arts college in Minnesota, I knew this would be a very different university experience.

Every fall, thousands of students overwhelm the city, ready to begin or continue their studies. The student body of the University of Leeds was bigger than the population of my hometown. From the first moment I stepped on campus, it seemed crowded and chaotic, and I felt very old. As a woman in her thirties who had had a career and completed two stints in the Peace Corps, I wasn't interested in going on pub crawls with teenagers. Instead, I set out to find the local lindy hoppers.

I really hoped I would be able to locate at least a few fellow lindy hop enthusiasts in Leeds. At that point in my life social dancing had become my primary social activity; I wasn't sure if I remembered how to make friends any other way.

When I looked at the facts, I felt optimistic. Leeds, one of the biggest cities in England, had a massive student population. Surely, there would be a lindy hop community here.

Finding that community proved difficult, however. My initial online search revealed a basic website advertising an outdated class series. When I emailed the local instructors, no one returned my messages. I waited, and finally, at the end of September, I saw an announcement on the website that the classes were restarting.

The first class was in the basement of a sports bar. With bad lighting and low ceilings, it was a far cry from the grand ballrooms I'd frequented in Seattle. Luckily, the community made up for it. Everyone was friendly, welcoming, and delighted to have a new, experienced lindy hopper in the scene. They all wanted to dance. Before I left that night, the instructors invited me to teach future classes.

The next week, I was first to arrive. Jo, one of the organizers I'd met the week before, walked in a few minutes later and introduced his friend, Rob. Rob was slender, looked to be in his early 20s, and had dark hair and thick glasses.

"You've got to dance with this girl!" Jo told Rob. "We need to get her teaching as soon as possible."

I chatted with Rob briefly. He seemed confident and intellectual, and I learned he had recently graduated from the University of Leeds with a degree in philosophy. He now worked for his dad as a medical sales representative and was one of the main lindy hop teachers in town.

Rob quickly became one of my most influential mentors. He and the other teachers believed in my potential as an instructor, despite the awkwardness of my first classes. In Seattle, I'd been an avid social dancer with no interest in teaching. Because of that, I'd never thought about how to describe what I was doing or how moves worked. Teaching required me to translate what I felt into coherent directions for others.

Although this was a challenge, I stuck with the process. With limited opportunities for social dancing in Leeds, I wanted another fulfilling way to grow my abilities as a dancer. In the following months, I honed my teaching skills by accepting every class offered to me. I would spend long hours preparing, and always asked for feedback from my students and fellow instructors. By taking classes as a leader and trying out my skills with the follows in the scene, I also learned how to teach both roles.

Performing was another thing I hadn't explored much, so I joined an annual lindy hop performance fundraiser. Over the holidays, we danced all day for crowds of Christmas shoppers to raise money for charity. I made lots of friends through the event, and it quickly became one of my favorite holiday traditions.

Finally, I worked up the courage to host a weekly social dance. I missed the social dances back home and wanted to create more opportunities for lindy hoppers to hone their skills and enjoy time together. I scouted out a venue, created a logo, started collecting music, and learned to DJ.

Becoming more involved with the Leeds lindy hop scene meant spending more time with Rob. He was similarly passionate about dancing, and we often worked together on classes or events. As we got to know each other more, an attraction developed. We began flirting, and, on a few occasions, we kissed.

These sweet moments were not worth the feeling afterward. Each time, we immediately regretted the decision and swore it would never happen again. If we were to start dating, something could go wrong. There was a chance we might lose our friendship or create awkwardness on the dance scene. We both felt invested in creating a healthy, flourishing lindy hop community, not a community with romantic drama.

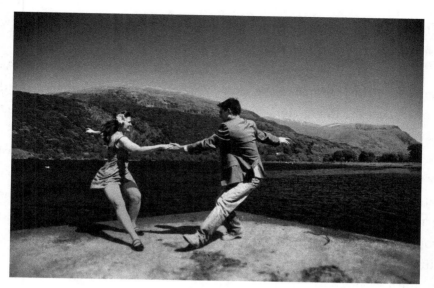

Tina and Rob dance lindy hop at Llanberis Lake in Snowdonia, Wales
Photo credit: Simon Shield

Even without romance, our relationship deepened. Rob and I were both at turning points in our lives. After years of traveling and adventure, I was ready to stay in one place. Rob wasn't passionate about medical sales and was trying to figure out his next move. I began to lean on him during challenging moments, and he did the same with me.

During one rough patch, when Rob needed a place to live, I tentatively suggested he stay at my house. As an introvert who deeply values alone time, I wasn't sure how this would go. I worried that spending too much time in close proximity to him would wear on me and challenge our friendship. To my surprise, though, I thoroughly enjoyed having Rob around. We danced, made meals together, talked for hours, and snuggled all the time. It felt like a sleepover.

Rob and I frequently discussed what he would do next. He was toying with the idea of being a full-time dance instructor, and began putting together a proposal to his parents for a business loan.

With each passing week, the line between friend and romantic partner became blurrier and blurrier. The occasional kissing returned.

When it was time for Rob to move, we were closer than ever. His new apartment became my second home.

One night, Rob invited his brother Jeff and me over for dinner. As the better cook, I prepared the meal. We had a lovely time chatting and showing Jeff the interesting features of Rob's new place. Everything felt easy and comfortable.

After dinner, Jeff left, and I stayed behind to help clean up. As we washed dishes and wiped down the table, we talked about how connected we'd become. It had seemed obvious that I would be at the apartment for his brother's first visit. It had been equally clear that I would be the hostess. We began to wonder how things would be different if we were a couple. For all intents and purposes, we realized, we already were.

When we made our relationship official, no one was surprised.

Becoming a couple changed little between us, with one notable exception: our fights about dance intensified. We suddenly cared much more about what the other person thought. Now romantic partners, and with our lives increasingly intertwined, we both craved more approval from one another and developed a greater sensitivity to feedback. Because of this, constructive criticism became a danger zone.

Previously, when we had been just dance partners, feedback might have been met with slight annoyance. Now, however, it stung. Remarks felt more personal and intense. We increasingly desired validation from one another.

We argued about topics such as technique or methods for approaching a new idea in class. A small disagreement would quickly spiral into, "How can we even teach together if you think that!?"

Our fights continued to get worse until one pivotal weekend, when class planning devolved into an hour-long argument. Frustrated, we decided to give up. We needed time apart to cool off.

As I walked out the door, I remembered Rob hadn't had breakfast.

"I know you're angry with me," I said, "but please promise me you'll eat something, because I love you!"

It was the first time I'd said those words, and I remember being doubly shocked. I was surprised at what I'd just said, as well as at how I could still care so much about Rob while he was being a stubborn jackass. We went our separate ways, but Rob later shared how much the experience had meant to him. He appreciated that I could have such strong feelings of love right after a big argument.

This was a pivotal event for two reasons: we recognized the depth of our feelings for one another, and we became inspired to find better ways to address conflict. Supporting one another, we decided, was more important than being right.

We decided to do our best to avoid speaking in absolutes, to trust that there were multiple good options, and to assume that we both had a role in what went wrong. We would then each pick something to change in our own dancing or behavior that could have been at the root of the challenge. We shared with one another what the change would be, and then put it into action. Through this approach, our disagreements became less common and less fierce.

I felt inspired by how we worked through the conflict, and charmed that dance had given me an avenue to become the best version of myself. More than ever, I found myself appreciating the community and opportunity that lindy hop had brought to my life.

A year after Rob and I officially started dating, my visa was due to expire. With few full-time job prospects and little hope of obtaining a work visa as a freelance theatre practitioner and dance instructor, it was time to make some big decisions. Just before Christmas, I pitched an idea to Rob.

"I know this is a crazy idea, but what if we got married?"

Neither of us had had marriage in our life plans. We both thought of it as a bureaucratic formality, rather than an important event. In this case, it was a means to an end: a way to stay together and continue the life we loved.

A month later, we got married in a small, unassuming room at the Leeds Town Hall. Everything about the day was simple and lovely. I wore a dress I'd purchased for £18; we danced to a playlist of our favorite music, and Rob's mum ordered a cake from the local bakery.

On the way to our wedding lunch with Rob's family, we posted my visa application two days ahead of the deadline. In the coming days, we would be surprised by how marriage had changed us. The experience felt less like a formality and more like a real, lifelong commitment.

***

Our commitment to each other, as well as to the lindy hop community, continues today. We've established a dance company; we continue to run classes and events, and we have taught at workshops across the UK. We've also made guest appearances on *Peaky Blinders*, as well as a few other English television shows. Our scene has grown, and, four years after our marriage, we welcomed Leeds' newest (and tiniest) dancer: our daughter Talia.

Talia began dancing long before she was born. I danced with her in my belly, and even in the delivery room as we waited for her arrival. She's become a regular at our classes, where I've taught while I carried her in a sling or she played in the corner. Talia loves jazz music, is learning steps, and repeats the phrases she hears us say often in class. Rob and I joke she'll replace us by the time she's three.

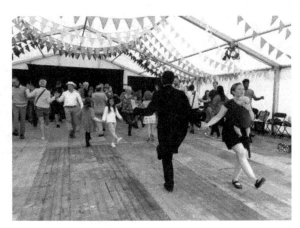

Rob and Tina teach lindy hop at the Underneath the Stars Festival in Yorkshire, England, with baby Talia
Photo credit: Steph Birks-Thelier

While lindy hop started as a hobby, it became my North Star. It showed me the way to community in Leeds, as well as the many other places I lived and visited. The dance also catalyzed more compassion in my relationship with Rob, and will be something we will always share.

These days, I'm able to watch the ways in which lindy hop plays an important role in others' lives, as well as my own. Our students regularly tell stories about how this dance has changed their lives: lovely couples have met in our classes; painfully shy people have become kick-ass performers, and a few students have become international instructors. Many others have found friendship, acceptance, and a much-needed release through this nurturing dance tradition.

Lindy hop continues to inspire me to learn and grow. Lately, I've focused on learning more about the social context of lindy hop and other Black dances from the early 20th century, which is enriching my experience as a dancer. Hopefully, it's also making me a better steward of this dance that I love. While I can never replace some of the incredible teachers I learned from, such as Frankie Manning and Dawn Hampton, I will do my best to share lindy hop with my community in a way that celebrates the magnitude of this Black American dance tradition.

Recommended resources:

Gould, M. (2020, July 07). Frankie Manning Foundation. Retrieved July 12, 2020, from https://www.frankiemanningfoundation.org/

Miller, N. (2010). *Swing Baby Swing!* San Francisco, CA: Blurb Books.

Shield, T. (n.d.). Swing Dance Leeds. Retrieved July 08, 2020, from http://swingdanceleeds.com/

White, B. (2011, February 22). An Index of Basic Classic Clips.

Retrieved July 07, 2020, from
https://www.google.co.uk/amp/s/swungover.wordpress.com/2011/0
2/22/an-index-of-basic-classic-clips/amp/

PART 3: UNEXPECTED OPPORTUNITIES

"It is strange, but true, that the most important turning points of life often come at the most unexpected times and in the most unexpected of ways."
—Napoleon Hill

Beyond your best-laid plans, adventure awaits. In fact, sometimes saying "Yes!" to new or spontaneous opportunities is the path to your most epic dance experiences. As the authors in this section head into unknown territory, you'll see how they challenge their assumptions and more deeply connect with the local culture and people.

DANCING IN THE DUNES

Alex Milewski

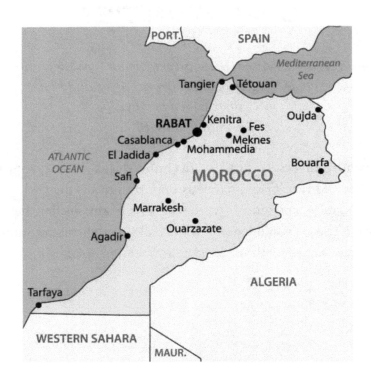

About the author: Alex is a full-time movement artist and educator based out of Boulder, Colorado, USA. He began breaking (breakdancing) in 2005, when he went to a class and was subsequently invited to practice with Denver-based crew Get Wit This (GWT), the most renowned Colorado crew at the time. Alex's main teachers in GWT were Fate, Dash, and Eppie.

Alex's mentors made a point to teach him about the roots of breaking. They wanted him to know about the original breakers and the culture of the community, especially because he was the only white kid on the crew at the time.

In the following years, Alex would travel with his crewmates to visit important breaking landmarks around the United States, such as 1520 Sedgwick Avenue in New York, where Kool Herc held the original house parties that set the groundwork for hip hop culture. During these trips, he also studied with original breakers such as Ken Swift, Crazy Legs, KujoIvan, and Storm.

In 2008, Alex moved from Denver to Boulder, Colorado, where he started his crew, Worm Tank, and later co-founded Block1750, a dance-based community center that provides an artistic home for people of all ages and backgrounds.

Alex's dancing is rooted in breaking, tricking, contemporary, house dance, and krump. When he moves, he focuses on improv, musicality, and expression. He travels often to share his experience and art with communities around the globe.

Our story begins with an artistic collaboration between two characters: an American breaker and a Senegalese singer. I, the breaker (or "b-boy,"[9] as male breakdancers are called), was traveling solo through Morocco to surf, experience the country, and, of course, dance.

Before I'd left Boulder, Colorado, a Moroccan friend of mine had recommended I visit Essaouira during my trip. Grateful for this tip, I added it to my itinerary. Essaouira is a coastal port city a few hours west of Marrakesh by rickety bus. A laid-back location with just 80,000 inhabitants, it's a nice break from the busy streets of larger, more touristy cities nearby. During the day, you drink sweet Moroccan mint tea while watching waves break against the city's tall, stone walls. It's often breezy, given the strong Alizee trade winds, so it's a popular location for surfing, windsurfing, and kitesurfing. Head down to the sandy beach, and you'll almost always find someone getting ready to play in the sea.

On my first day in town, I made my way to the medina. Medinas are old, charismatic parts of town, full of beautiful architecture and always bustling with vendors selling goods such as dates, spices, and olives. You walk through narrow streets lined with carpets for sale, and sometimes glimpse the interior of mosques where Muslims go to pray five times each day. The air is alive with the smells of argan oil and incense.

Essaouira's medina includes a large, open square. After a long travel day, I was itching to move my body. The square seemed like an ideal place to dance, so I set up my speaker and started to groove.[10] As a b-boy, my groove involves warming up with toprocks. This foundational move in breaking involves rhythmic footwork and is typically the first thing breakers learn when they begin to dance. I also

---

[9] Within the breakdance community, "b-boy" is more often spelled without the hyphen.

[10] One of the editors pointed out that I did not first look to make sure dancing in this square was culturally appropriate. This was eye-opening to me, and has taught me more about how to be a responsible traveler by being conscious of my visitor status in communities and cultures that are not my own.

got my upper body moving with handstands and other upside-down balances known as freezes.[11]

A few minutes later, a tall Black man in a brown business suit and cowboy hat set up an amp nearby. He started playing instrumental music from his phone and singing in a beautiful, slow-flowing voice.

Naturally, I turned off my speaker and started to dance to his music. Our impromptu collaboration began to attract attention. People watched and filmed as we played off each other's energy and wove our artistry together. At the end of a series of songs, when I was too exhausted to dance any more, I walked over to the musician and thanked him for his music. He gave me a huge, warm smile and complimented my dancing and spirit. He was a musician from Senegal, he told me.

Since arriving in Morocco, I'd met many Senegalese people, and learned that the Senegalese are one of Morocco's most populous migrant communities. After chatting a little with my new musician friend, I said goodbye and began to head out of the medina.

This is when two short Moroccan men approached me shyly. In their late teens or early 20s, they were wearing basic Western clothing and carrying small backpacks.

"Hey," they said in their Moroccan accents. "Where you from?"

"I'm from Colorado in the United States," I said.

"How long dancing?"

"About 11 years," I replied.

I didn't speak Arabic, and their English was limited, so the next part of our conversation involved lots of gesturing. Ten minutes later, I was pretty sure they were also b-boys, that there would be a practice that night in a place outside the medina, and that I was supposed to meet them back at the square at 6 p.m. so I could attend.

***

---

[11] Visit @dancetravelabroad to see the videos of Alex in action in the medina.

151

When I showed up that evening, I was nervous. While I had a cardinal rule about dancing – if an opportunity arises, I take it – I also knew it was a risk to go off on an adventure at night in a foreign country with people I'd never met.[12]

Despite my concerns, I was excited, too. I'd never met Moroccan b-boys. If these guys were, in fact, a part of the community, I trusted that our shared love of dance would unite us, and that I would have an incredible opportunity to check out the b-boy scene in Essaouira.

The two young men showed up in the square right on time, and this time I got their names: Yassine and Adil. Even though they were short (most b-boys are, so that was a good sign), they didn't dress like the other breakers I'd met during my travels.

Breaking culture in the United States, as well as in most other developed countries, has its own swagger and unofficial dress code. Most breakers wear Adidas or Dickies pants, Puma shoes, and some sort of windbreaker jacket. These guys were just wearing sweatpants and normal t-shirts. It wasn't until later that I learned Moroccan breakers aren't identified by what they wear on the outside so much as what they have on the inside. I now know that this can be said for many dancers in developing countries around the world, including Mexico, Colombia, Ecuador, Indonesia, and Thailand.

I find this incredibly refreshing: one reason that dancing is so beautiful is its integrity. Someone can either do a move, or they cannot. You don't need to have $200 sneakers to be a dope breaker; you just need to break.

As we walked toward the outskirts of the city, Yassine took out his phone and showed me videos of an up-and-coming Moroccan b-boy named Simocroc. I had never heard of him, but he was incredibly skilled and moving in ways I had never seen before. This put me at ease for a

---

[12] Looking back, I know that being able to take this risk was part of my privilege as a white American man. My b-girl friends may not have been comfortable doing something similar, and I imagine that someone of a different skin color or ethnicity would have less confidence in the local authorities being on their side.

while, but as we ventured further out of the city, I began to worry again. We were far away from the area of town I knew, and I still had no solid proof that these guys were breakers.

My heart was beating fast when we arrived at a small, circular amphitheater beside a busy three-way intersection. The floor was black-and-white marble arranged in a design that looked like the inside of a compass.

"This is our spot!" announced Yassine and Adil.

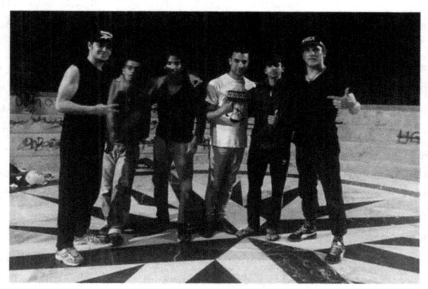

From left to right: Yassine, Mhmoud, Adil,
another dancer, Younes, and Alex
Photo credit: Anonymous

While I have been to hundreds of practice spaces around the world, this was by far the wildest training spot I'd seen. Not only were there breakers getting down and spectators watching from the surrounding seating, but there were also rollerblading kids zooming in and out of the amphitheater and grabbing onto cars heading through the busy three-way intersection. I wasn't sure how the breakers could concentrate with everything going on.

The scene was impressive, and yet there was still a cherry on top:

behind the dance area was a massive open desert with—get this—camel parking. After a day of toting tourists around the beach, this was where the camel riders came to leave their animals for the evening. So, in addition to the noise of traffic and music, you would often hear a camel grunt.

***

I had come to Essaouira expecting to stay for a few days. Three weeks later, I was still there, enjoying dancing with the local b-boys. After that first night, I had immediately become part of the family. We would go to the beach to work on flips every day, and meet at the practice spot at 7 p.m. almost every evening. Other nights, we would head to a martial arts gym to try new moves on a padded floor. This is where I met another one of the b-boys, Mhmoud. While Adil, Yassine, and I had shared the language of dance since we met, Mhmoud made the language barrier between all of us less of a hurdle. He would translate between English and Arabic for us all, making sure we were all on the same page about communication, planning, and – more than a few times – joking.

As we continued to dance together, I discovered that the b-boys were also accomplished capoeiristas. Capoeira, an Afro-Brazilian martial art that combines elements of dance, acrobatics, and music, requires strength, skill, and discipline.

"Who taught you all this?" I asked one day after learning some capoeira from them on the beach.

"Nobody taught us," Mhmoud replied. "We just saw it on YouTube and started to play."

This was my first glimpse of what it means to be a b-boy from the inside out. These guys were thirsty for knowledge, as well as committed to developing skills no matter the circumstances. I found this to be extremely empowering; skills and perseverance say way more than shoes, shirts, or jackets. This was true with the original breakers, too, as the dance began with young people in the Bronx who were hungry to learn, to do the next "crazy move," and to be the best they could be.

Seeing my new friends' talent also challenged one of my long-held assumptions, which was that you need a teacher to improve. This is not true at all, I realized. You can simply seek inspiration and try whatever you want. This felt like an access point to a new level of freedom in my own learning.

Previously, I had worried that this sort of copycat skills development would be considered irreverent. In fact, this was something that my earliest teachers had taught me not to do. In breaking, we call copying a skill from someone else "biting," and it is heavily frowned upon.

Now, I saw that this belief had caused me to miss out on a powerful way to develop new skills and ideas. These b-boys weren't being disrespectful. Without local teachers available, they were using videos to develop the skills required to invent brand-new signature moves.

One evening, my friends asked me if I would be interested in going with them to Canada. I was confused at first, thinking they were talking about Canada, the country, but it became clear the location was not too far from town. I was in!

On Saturday morning, we traveled one hour out of the city by local "bus" (a converted cargo van with benches and chairs to seat eight – or, in Morocco, 18 – people). We got off the bus in the middle of nowhere: a completely unmarked section of desert with nothing but sand as far as the eye could see. I was glad I trusted these guys by that point.

We had walked 45 minutes into the desert when we came upon a small oasis. Until then, I hadn't thought oases were real. I was delighted! Right in the middle of this inhospitable-looking landscape was a small stream running next to palm trees and green grass. The area was about half the size of a soccer field, and it was home to many species of plants and insects. Life thrived here, and the greenery could be seen following the stream into the distance.

The b-boys began settling in, unloading fresh veggies, dry rice, and bread from their backpacks.

"We have pots here," said Adil.

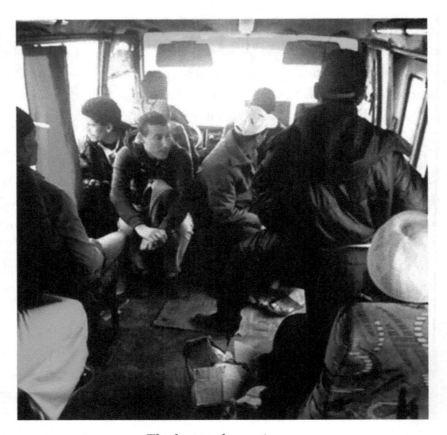

The bus to the oasis
Photo credit: Alex Milewski

He headed over to a palm tree and began to walk slowly back out into the desert. It took me a few moments to realize he was counting his steps—actually *pacing out* a distance from the tree (talk about some real buried treasure vibes!). He then stopped and began to dig with his hands. Out of the sand came cooking pots, matches, and everything else we would need to cook the meal.

We gathered water from the stream, built a fire, and chopped up our vegetables. We would be preparing a *tajine*, a traditional Moroccan dish named after the earthenware pot in which it is cooked. We put the vegetables, along with salt, pepper, turmeric, and other spices, in the bottom section of the tajine and covered it with the tajine's circus-tent-shaped top.

We spent the next three hours tumbling on the sand, climbing trees, and jumping off tires that the b-boys had dragged into the desert. I then had one of the best meals of my life. We ate the tajine from a single dish with our hands. The flavors were bold, and the aromas of fresh cooked onions, peppers, zucchini, eggplant, carrots, couscous, and spices filled the air.

As we ate, I asked Mhmoud why they called the oasis "Canada."

"Our friend who discovered this place always wanted to go to Canada," he responded. "We call it Canada because it's far away from town, just like the real Canada."

As crazy as it sounds, I had a Canadian flag patch in my backpack, which I had intended to bring home to sew onto a travel jacket I was making. I found some wire in my pack and mounted the patch on a nearby tree, happy to make a small contribution to this magical place.

As we were walking back to the road just before sunset, Adil pointed into the distance.

"Beautiful, you see?"

I looked and saw blue skies as far as the horizon.

"Yes, the sky is beautiful." I agreed, pausing for a moment to take it in. But then Adil gestured again, laughing.

"You see the water?"

As I looked closer, I realized it wasn't all blue skies. The color of the sky and sea were so closely matched that I hadn't noticed the ocean at all. It was a sight I will never forget.

Once back at the main road, we waited for the bus to arrive. By the time it did, the sun had almost set, and the stars were just becoming visible over the sand dunes. Driving back through the wide expanse of desert into Essaouira, I felt a pang of gratitude for the Senegalese man in the medina. He'd played the music; I had danced, and these new, amazing friends found me.

There is so much connection and beauty to be found across the world, and you never know when or where it will appear. It could be staring at you from behind a fruit stall or across a plaza. As we travel and dance, we have an obligation to our one precious life: to consciously choose when to throw caution, old stories, and technique to the wind in order to just live. By finding the courage to express ourselves and connect with others, we can turn our dream of exciting new adventures into reality.

Recommended resources:

Lee, B. (Director). (2017). *Planet B-Boy* [Video file]. USA: Elephant Eye Films.

Sjoberg, A. (Director), Sjoberg, A. (Writer), & Jones, N., Tabibian, S., Lippke, I., Lippke, A., Millsap, R., Gomez, M. P., . . . Galloway, L. (Producers). (2015). *Shake the Dust* [Video file]. USA: Bond/360.

CUBA'S WELCOME EMBRACE

Nneya Richards

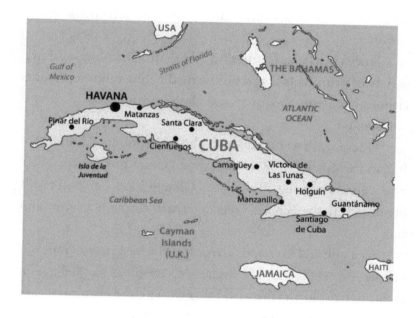

About the author: Multi-hyphenate Nneya Richards is a journalist and public speaker who began her career at 16 as a founding contributing editor to *Teen Vogue* magazine. She is frequently featured in travel and fashion publications, including *Condé Nast Traveler*, *Vogue*, and *Vice*. Nneya is the founder of *'N A Perfect World*, a curated intersection of travel, food, style, and geopolitics inspired by the millennial global citizen.

Nneya has been featured in *Forbes*, on *CBS News*, and in a variety of print, video, and online media. She often represents airlines, tourism boards, and hotel groups as a brand ambassador.

Nneya was recently honored by the National Chamber of Italian Fashion as a Digital Creative of Color to Know in 2020. She serves on the board of Glam4Good, a non-profit organization that creates social impact through beauty and style.

As a cultural exchange advocate, Nneya aims to empower people—especially BIPOC women—to travel, as she believes it is through exploring the world that we will bridge cultural gaps and misunderstandings. We are all ambassadors.

The question I am asked most often as a travel writer is, "What is your favorite country to visit?" Like a parent being quizzed as to which is her favorite child, I'm reluctant to say, citing unfairness to other locales. That said, I'll share a secret with you: I do have a preferred five, and they have something in common.

My wholehearted love of each of these destinations developed based on how I embraced the culture and how the culture, in turn, embraced me. This connection often came unexpectedly. It was sometimes simple, such as hearing someone say, "Hey, are you hungry?" Other times, it was grandiose, like being pulled up on stage at a music festival.

As a writer who is used to documenting much of my travels for public consumption, these sweet moments are the ones that I squirrel away just for me, guarding them as I would the privacy of my loved ones. I sometimes dance around these experiences to color my travel tales, but I never share the intimate details.

For you, however, I'll share how Cuba became one of my favorite locations and what made me want to go back. The story begins in my early years, as I slowly learned about the country.

Initially, my knowledge about Cuba was limited. Although my paternal grandmother was born in Cuba, I did not grow up immersed in Cuban culture. My mother hails from a family of proud Jamaicans, and this is the culture that has shaped my entire life—in addition to American customs, obviously. Therefore, neither familial ties nor my time growing up in New York City (where, due to immigration patterns, other Latinx island peoples like Puerto Ricans and Dominicans are more heavily represented) exposed me to a great deal of Cuban culture.

Nonetheless, the more I learned about Cuba – whether through Cuban-American friends, history class, or pop culture – the more I felt drawn to the country. Knowing it was so close to the United States, but that it was forbidden to visit, made it all the more alluring.

This is why I was so excited when, in December 2014, President Barack Obama and Cuban President Raúl Castro announced they would start normalizing relations between the United States and Cuba.

161

Immediately, my mother and I began making our plans for a four-day, four-night trip to the country. We would arrive in August 2015, a few months ahead of when President Obama would become the first US president to visit Cuba since 1928.

***

What you rarely see in movies or read about in travelogues is the moment someone arrives in the airport of a new place. Often, it's not sexy. There are fluorescent lights, people who are tired and irritable after long flights and customs lines, and the advertisements and installations that the country's tourism industry uses to grab your attention.

In some countries, singing men or women playing the harp greet you at the airport. Cuba didn't have this pomp and circumstance. Landing in Havana, my travel-weary mother and I were greeted only by sunshine, blue skies, and palm trees surrounding the runway. The humid, briny Caribbean air revitalized us. We were island girls, after all.

Even though José Martí International Airport did not have a welcome band, it certainly had a rhythm that caught you and set you in tune with the island. The roll of the luggage on Havana's airport linoleum made a noise like maracas; the greeting of a long-awaited relative sounded like a song. Suitcases crashed against the bottoms of trunks like Bantu bongos. The sun-kissed Cubans' swaying hips and melodic speech hinted at the island's love for *son cubano* music and the Afro-Cuban *rumba*.

Many people talk about Havana as if it's a city frozen in time. While there are things that harken back to the 1950s – such as the restored, bubblegum-pink Cadillacs I passed outside a mint-green mansion my first day – I found the city to be alive and dynamic with music, dancing, and art.

In a way, this felt normal to me. Dancing and music are part of my Jamaican family's cultural inheritance. Only recently, after talking to white American friends or those from European backgrounds, did I think, "Oh, it isn't the norm to have a sound system and dance contest at a two-year-old's birthday party?"

In Jamaican culture, a sound system is an institution, with stacks of speakers, turntables, and a generator morphing into a Transformers-like figure that is set up for parties at which DJs, sound engineers, and MCs battle for musical supremacy.

Sometime in early childhood, those backyard dance contests had sparked a desire in me for more formal dance training. This is how I ended up taking ballet, tap, and modern dance classes in my younger years. I also became an appreciator of Cuban dance forms thanks to my New York City school's partnership with Ballet Hispánico, an American dance company based in NYC whose mission is to celebrate and explore Latinx cultures through dance training, innovative performance, and community engagement. Later, in college at Amherst, I would continue my artistic education through courses in theatre and dance.

These experiences all fostered my appreciation for the performing arts. For this reason, while in Cuba, I hoped to see Cuban dance, and *perhaps* attend a Cuban dance performance. Still, this wouldn't be something my mother and I actively sought out. When we plan our mother-daughter trips, we always leave room for the unexpected. Since I write about off-the-beaten-path experiences, I thrive off local recommendations and like to have time in my itinerary for spontaneity.

✳✳✳

One of the few things on our schedule was volunteering at the Muraleando Community Arts Center in the Lawton area of Havana. Between 1999 and 2019, Americans were allowed to travel to Cuba on a "people-to-people" visa that permitted visits to the country for cultural and educational activities. Going to Cuba, therefore, was not to be a beach vacation, or even solely an opportunity to take in the sights and sounds. Volunteering had to be a part of the itinerary, and so I was happy to find that the Muraleando Arts Center, which provided music and fine arts classes to local children, was accepting assistants.

Early one morning, we hopped into a taxi and headed to Lawton,

163

carrying our donation of supplies. We were unsure what we would be doing, as our Muraleando contact, Jesús, had kept it vague.

"We would be delighted for you to come volunteer!" he'd said over email, but he had not provided any more details.

As the taxi turned the final corner, we were welcomed by the sounds of a percussion band. We saw kids playing in the streets, clowns, and even someone on stilts. Everything was a visual feast! The community arts center (a repurposed water tank) and the streets surrounding it were beautifully decorated by Cuban artists who had used every shade on the color wheel for painted murals, mosaic tile work, and sculptural art made from reclaimed materials like bathtubs and car parts. The setting evoked a major motion picture studio's wonderland set, and music and laughter were the soundtrack to the scene.

That day, the center was holding a party to celebrate the end of the summer programs and the beginning of the school year. We explored the facility with Jesús, who gave us an overview of Muraleando's impact on the community and lit up as he talked about current and past students.

"So many people in our community take pride in this center," he said, looking out at the dozens of children playing. "It gives the young people learning opportunities in the fine arts that they may not have otherwise have due to family income or circumstances. It's a project of love for all of us."

We would not be volunteering with a class, we found out, as today was all about celebrating. Our time would instead be spent enjoying this day with the Muraleando community—an experience that would introduce us to many students and local artisans. That morning, my mother and I met many people and shopped for paintings and jewelry at a pop-up the artisans had set up in a classroom.

At a certain point, we settled in for a performance from an amazing local son band, Mambu & Company. The vocalist's soulful rendition of "Quizás" had my mother and me swaying in our seats. With her blue-and-white-striped pants and her dyed red afro, the singer was a star:

Afro-Cuban beauty personified.

As the band switched to a percussion-heavy rumba, a young boy of no more than six commanded center stage. Wearing a turquoise Muraleando graphic t-shirt, shorts, and black high-tops, this young man looked like any other kid his age, but when he danced, *wow*. Back straight, his moves precise yet fluid as he sang along with the band, he carried himself with the professionalism of a dancer decades his senior.

Although this boy was a dance student at Muraleando, he was about to become my teacher. My mom and I sat in our chairs, tapping our feet in an attempt to mirror him, while at times taking video of his performance. Most of those videos came out horribly shaky, though, since we couldn't help but dance. One chorus in, he glided toward us and took my hand. He wanted me to join him!

Nervous, but full of excitement, I shoved my recording camera and my phone into my mother's lap. I had anticipated *watching* a performance, not dancing myself!

Despite my aforementioned love of dance, choreography has never come easily to me, and I've never trained with a partner. The few times I've danced with talented leads, I've become flustered, feeling like a mere ornament, and a dull one at that.

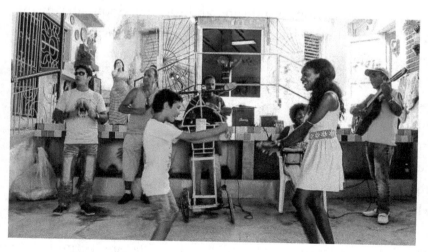

Nneya dances at Muraleando with the young man
Photo credit: Heather Walker

Maybe it was the shouts of encouragement or the considerate, patient nature of my young dance partner, but I was not rattled this time. As the young man demonstrated shoulder shakes and floor rolls for me to imitate, all while smiling and singing, I found myself able to copy him on the same feet that typically get tangled when I'm trying to learn TikTok choreography.

After a minute or so, a female clown joined us. Only upon seeing my teacher's eyes light up and hearing him giggle with the appearance of this unexpected guest did I   remember his age. This moment was bliss: the young boy was smiling at the clown and dancing; my mother was half out of her seat, recording video and cheering, and I was somehow executing new dance moves to live music. Suddenly, I was no longer just a spectator. Here, amongst these Cuban performers, I had become part of the tableau.

"The idea of the starving artist is foreign in Cuba," Jesús told us afterward. "While the country may not have thrived financially as it could have due to economic sanctions by the United States, the Cuban system makes way for dignity in community-building professions."

After Fidel Castro took over the country in 1959, he began to implement his vision of rebuilding Cuba as a Communist country with access for all to education, healthcare, and the arts. Soon after, many government-funded art schools such as the Escuela Nacional de Arte emerged, offering training in visual and performing arts for people of every socioeconomic background.

Later, in the Special Period, Castro allowed artists to travel abroad to promote and sell their work, recognizing that the art community that he himself had put on a pedestal had the potential to generate revenue for the island from other countries. In giving artists this special privilege, Castro provided the US and other foreign countries access to Cuban art, which was and still is wildly successful. Many Cuban artists enjoy these prerogatives to this day. While most private sector jobs are controlled by the government, successful artists are permitted to participate in other economies.

Today, as a result of these policies, Cuba's artistic contributions are recognized worldwide. The roots of salsa music, for instance, originated in Eastern Cuba from the Cuban son and Afro-Cuban rumba. Beginning in the 1920s, as American jazz gained popularity all over the world, jazz rhythms were infused into the music as well. Cuba's dance traditions – specifically the casino, mambo, and pachanga – also played a critical role in the development of salsa dancing, which was primarily created by Puerto Ricans in New York City in the 1960s as a combination of Cuban dances and American jazz moves.

***

After a few hours, we said goodbye to Jesús and the other members of the Muraleando community, thanking them for a beautiful experience. My mother and I then left to explore the Malecon (the broad esplanade that lines Havana's coast) and went to a landmark spot, the Hotel Habana Riviera, for an afternoon drink. My mother had a mojito, while I delighted in a Cuba libre: a Coke mixed with Cuban rum. The buzz of the spirits only added to our bubbliness after the morning of dance at Muraleando.

As we exited the hotel, a tall, smiling gentleman standing in front of a horse and carriage tipped his fedora to us. My mother and I waved back and continued on our way. We didn't have a plan; we were just meandering with no specific destination in mind. When we began taking photos in front of a vintage gold Cadillac, however, we outed ourselves as foreigners. The gentleman, realizing we were not Cubans but Black Americans, came over to us.

"I don't see a lot of Afro-American tourists!" he said. "Where are you from?"

"New York!" we told him.

"I'm Julio, and I will show you the true Havana," he said, offering us a hand up into the carriage.

While this might have been his pitch to everyone, we began to truly believe Julio after he took us to his home, the local ration market where he bought groceries, and many Afro-Cuban haunts in the city.

As we made our way through Havana's neighborhoods, Julio told us about his time in Australia wrestling for Cuba's national team, and gave us his candid take on the Cuban government.

One of our final stops was a popular tourist spot, El Floridita Bar in Havana's historic district. This venue is known for being a part of *Hemingway's Havana*, and even has a bronze statue of the literary great sitting at his favorite place at the bar. Julio asked if we wanted a famous daiquiri, but by now the mojito from Habana Riviera had started to affect my mom, who rarely drinks.

"I'm fine," she said in a sing-song voice as she tapped her toes to a live band playing in the corner of the restaurant. I nudged her with my shoulder, and we smiled. I began practicing the shoulder shake I'd learned just a few hours before, and my mom nodded along enthusiastically to the beats, her eyes closed.

I could tell she was really feeling the music, and so could Julio, apparently.

Suddenly, he took her hands and led her into the middle of the floor in that crowded bar. There, they began to dance a salsa/two-step hybrid! I couldn't remember the last time I'd seen my mom partner dance. Her pure, unadulterated joy was clear as she smiled and laughed, throwing her head back with abandon and never missing a beat. My mom and Julio were the only ones dancing. In that moment, my mom became a part of the tableau, just as I had at Muraleando.

We spent the rest of the afternoon with Julio. After lunch, he took us to a space where the Buena Vista Social Club - an ensemble of Cuban musicians established in 1996 to revive the music of pre-revolutionary Cuba - would be performing that evening. My mother and I purchased tickets for dinner and a show.

That night, dressed to the nines, we reveled in son Cubano music and dancing. The audience seemed to be mainly tourists, who would often excitedly rush toward the stage to film the performers. My mother and I did the same, though we spent the majority of our time dancing at our table, only pausing for sustenance when the band went on break between acts.

We hadn't expected that we would be immersed in Cuban music and dancing from morning to night that day, nor did we anticipate the final artistic surprise the city would offer us later in the trip.

***

One afternoon toward the end of our visit, my mother and I were walking in the neighborhood of Vedado, the site of many former embassies that had been remodeled into public spaces or homes for multiple Cuban families after the revolution. Suddenly, the quiet of the residential street was broken by the sonorous chords of a piano.

Peeking through the open, lattice-work gates of one of the buildings, we saw elegant dancers gliding across a ballroom that had been converted into a dance studio. This stately manor, it turned out, was the Cuban National Ballet School, the training center for one of the most prestigious dance companies in the world.

The entryway, festooned with bougainvilleas whose vines reached out to greet visitors, afforded us the perfect spot for an intimate viewing. The dancers' form was so perfect and their movements so precise that they seemed otherworldly.

After a few minutes, a member of the corps looked our way and winked. Feeling like we'd been discovered, my mother and I smiled shyly and pranced away, sashaying down the middle of the street to the notes of the piano.

***

These are the unexpected moments that bring Cuba to the forefront of my mind when I'm asked about my favorite destinations. There, dancing was what forged my connection to the culture.

For many, this country evokes the vision of a vintage postcard. But that time-capsule idea of Cuba is just a beautiful backdrop to the vibrant Havana of today that embraced my mother and me. My Cuba is alive and rooted in the present, a dynamic place where I've created treasured memories.

Recommended resources:

Associated Press. (2015, June 10). Cuban Artists Rolling in Foreign Money, Thanks to Topsy-Turvy Laws. Retrieved July 06, 2020, from https://www.billboard.com/articles/business/6590843/cuban-artists-rolling-in-foreign-money-thanks-to-topsy-turvy-laws

Ballet Hispanico. (2020). Retrieved July 06, 2020, from https://www.ballethispanico.org/

Ballet Nacional de Cuba. (n.d.). [Spanish only]. Retrieved July 06, 2020, from http://www.balletcuba.cult.cu/es

Broughton, S., Ellingham, M., & Trillo, R. (1999). *World Music: The Rough Guide* (p. 488). London, UK: Rough Guides.

Hernandez-Reguant, A. (Ed.). (2016). *Cuba in the Special Period: Culture and Ideology in the 1990s.* New York, NY: Palgrave Macmillan.

Juliao, D. (n.d.). Salsa Dance: Origin, History & Steps – Video & Lesson Transcript. Retrieved July 06, 2020, from https://study.com/academy/lesson/salsa-dance-origin-history-steps.html#:~:text=Salsa%20originated%20in%20the%201900s,New%20York%20by%20Cuban%20musicians.

Proyecto Comunitario Muraleando. (n.d.). Retrieved July 06, 2020, from https://www.facebook.com/proyectomuraleando/

NOT A BI-RACIAL BALLERINA

Natalie Preddie

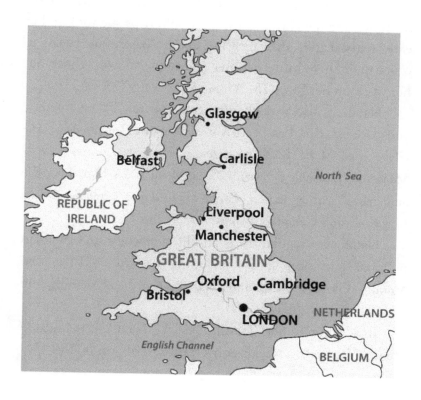

About the author: Canada-based Natalie Preddie is a mum to two beautiful little boys (with a new addition on the way) who already share her love of adventure. Natalie began documenting her travels during the solo trips she took in her early years. Later, after meeting her husband, she began to cover their shared international journeys. You can check out her work on her blog, *The Adventures of Natty P & Co.*

Natalie is also a sought-after travel writer, TV personality, and panelist. She has been featured in the *Toronto Star*, *The Globe and Mail*, *PAX Magazine*, *Travel + Leisure*, *BOLD Magazine*, *Ensemble Magazine*, *SavvyMom*, *CAA Magazine*, the *Sunwing Kidcation* expert panel, *TravelPulse Canada*, *Divine Magazine*, and *Canadian Family*.

Natalie is a regular travel and lifestyle guest on Canadian national television shows including *CityLine*, CTV's *Your Morning*, Global's *The Morning Show*, *Global News Morning*, and CHCH's *Morning Live*.

In addition to her "Travel Tuesday," Natalie is the host of *Moms in Reel Life*, a weekly conversation series on IGTV.

At the barre, I stared longingly into the mirror, wishing for any body other than the one I had. I focused on tucking in my round bum – a feature the really good dancers didn't seem to have – and trying to make my long arms appear graceful as they moved from position to position. No matter what I did, though, they just looked awkward. My disappointment in my physique didn't end there. Whenever I pulled my legs together, my muscular quads would flex instead of creating the perfect lines that were deemed ideal.

As a teenager, I wanted to be a ballet dancer, and I wanted it badly. This desire ate at my insides and gnawed at my brain. The dream of performing on stage for a company such as the National Ballet of Canada or the English National Ballet consumed me.

As a bi-racial teen in a primarily white dance community, I tried everything to be like my white ballerina friends. I learned the names of famous white dancers and watched ballets religiously. At night, I put weights on my toes to make my feet arch better, practiced exercises to try to shrink my bum, and toyed with ways to make my arms seem less angular. I also experimented with white hairstyles to make myself look more like my friends, who somehow always had the perfect slicked-back bun. Some of my attempts worked, while others ended up highlighting my frizz and curls. Despite all my efforts, the other dancers were just... better. In every possible way, they were better.

My high school dance teacher tried to free me, to help me see my beauty and my own unique potential. She told me to embrace the unique shape of my body. Still, I couldn't help but feel that doing this would symbolize an acceptance of defeat, sealing my fate as a non-ballerina.

The studio where I'd taken dance classes for years was known for its exceptional ballet tutelage. It continually produced award-winning dancers, and its graduates often became professional performers or received respected teaching positions. Those ballerinas were my idols: beautiful, thin, graceful, and yes, white.

At this studio, it was considered a huge accomplishment to complete your Royal Academy of Dance ballet exams, which were extremely difficult and had an abysmally low pass rate. Every movement, every musical count, and every breath was timed, judged, and graded.

Even though the odds were against me, I desperately wanted to complete my exams. After all, I knew the counts, I knew the steps, and I knew when to move my head to the left instead of the right. I practiced day in and day out at the studio, at home, and in any space where I could plié. My biggest struggle remained the one I was fighting against my own body: the way it wanted it to move and just be.

Every time my teacher would tell me that I wasn't ready for exam season, my heart would sink. A tear or two would fall as I stood alone in the studio after class, staring in the long mirror at the body that continually betrayed me. I would never be the ballerina I so desperately wanted to be.

***

By the time I was ready to graduate from high school, I felt more stuck than ever. Having not taken my ballet exams, I wasn't sure of what else to do to achieve my goal of becoming a ballerina. I had no support from anyone who looked or moved like me. What was next?

I decided I would enroll at a university and study media, information, and technology. It only took a few months there, however, before I realized that this wasn't my path. With no idea where I was going in life, I felt lost and afraid. My future seemed not just bleak, but non-existent.

I stopped dancing and fell into a deep depression that, after a few months, culminated in an attempt to take my own life. I took a few months to seek help, attempting to heal and grow, but I still had no sense of direction.

I slowly started to dance again at my local studio with the obscure intention to become a ballerina still floating somewhere in my head. During my depression, I had lost a significant amount of weight. Now, even though my round bum was gone, so were my passion and strength.

Every time I went to dance, I would wear a turtleneck sweater to hide the marks of self-harm on my arms and neck. Sometimes, I couldn't bring myself to practice. Instead, I would just sit in the empty studio, staring at my thin, ashen, fractured reflection. I struggled with my identity as a bi-racial woman, a dancer, a student, and even a human.

The next few months felt like mere emotionless survival. I floated from day to day in a haze.

Throughout that time, I continued to go to the studio, where I moved my body in new ways and worked on technique. Attempting to unwind the massive knot in my heart, I started seeing a therapist and a psychiatrist, and took time to read and journal. Little by little, the clouds seemed to break. Guided by my supportive parents, we created a safe space for me to heal, reflect, and imagine a future.

Later that year, when I felt I was ready to begin living again, I started auditioning for dance schools in London. My mother had been born and bred in England, and my family had spent a great deal of time there throughout my childhood and teenage years. I had always been enamored with that city: the sparkling lights, the living history, the glamour, and the 24/7 buzz of the metropolis. I would experience a physical rush - a tingle - when I landed at the airport, signifying that yes, this was where I was meant to be. Dancing in England's West End had been a dream of mine from the time I was a child, so it made sense for me to embark on the next chapter of my life there.

With painful anticipation, I waited for the rejection letters to arrive. Day after day, I watched the mailbox for any indication of my life's next step. Then it arrived: the piece of mail I had been waiting for—the one that could change my life. I held the envelope, hands shaking, breath held, both terrified and yearning to see what was inside.

Silently, I tore it open. I had been accepted to a dance school! Filled with fear, excitement, and disbelief, I readied myself for my studies. I pounded my pointe shoes, perfected my bun, and increased the weight on my toes to perfect my arch. *This time*, I was determined to get it right.

***

On my first day of school, with anxiety caught in my throat and my dance gear in a bag over my shoulder, I fumbled my way through registration and headed up to the main studio where the registrar would be giving a welcome speech.

As I sat down in the large hall, I started to look around, noticing the other students for the first time. Although it was a British school, the program attracted dancers from across the world, all eager for their moment in the spotlight. To my right, I saw a Black girl twiddling her thumbs nervously and tapping a beat with her heels on the wooden floor. To my left, an Asian girl was staring straight ahead, hands lying softly in her lap. In front of me, some boys were chatting excitedly among themselves. There were so many different types of people here: Black, Brown, white. This room held a breadth of beauty! Was this what dance looked like outside of my bubble?

Before I had time to ruminate on my new discovery, the program was underway. The Dean walked us through regular school protocols, rules, and expectations before introducing a dance number that would be performed by the school's third years.

As the dancers took the floor, my world began to spin. The group standing in front of me was an array of people of all colors. I saw hair like mine, not scraped back in a bun but free to fall, curl, and wind; there were also dreadlocks pulled back with scrunchies. Some of the performers had brown skin, round bums, angles, and curves. For the first time in a celebrated dance space, I was around people who looked like me.

I started to question everything I thought I knew about dance, my tiny world, and even myself. Was it possible for every body to move with grace, and for anyone to dance ballet? Could movement be an exploration, a sequence, a celebration? Was the world of dance as unforgiving as I had once believed, or was there room for "the other"?

And then the dancers on stage started to move.

They began with a traditional ballet, but without the "white-only" constrictions of strict lines and perfectly arched feet that I had come to recognize as the only way this dance could be done. And my goodness, it was beautiful.

The students performed with the grace, fluidity, and splendor that I knew ballet dancers to possess, but with bodies I hadn't known were allowed within the art form. Arms stretched beyond the constraints of strict lines; hips rolled to alternate rhythms, and feet flexed where I thought they could only point. Hair flipped and flowed, exaggerating the dancers' shapes. The corps shifted effortlessly from ballet to tap to modern dance before finally ending on a student-choreographed contemporary piece that combined all three.

This show was a celebration of camaraderie that honored the diversity, strength, and beauty of each dancer. As they spun and leapt across the floor, all the performers seemed genuinely happy, smiling and looking at each other as if to say, "I love what we are doing together."

For the first time, I could view my imperfections and failures as unique and magnificent advantages. I realized that I had spent too many years trying to contort my entire being into a small-town mold that simply didn't fit, and living in ignorance of a space that celebrated bodies like mine.

Here in this new world of dance, I saw my place. The more the students moved, the more at peace I felt. The anguish, self-doubt, and pain of my prior years slowly faded away. I was not alone.

Recommended resources:

Dance Spirit. (2020, June 04). Meet 10 Up-and-Coming Black Ballerinas Carrying on Misty Copeland's Message of Diversity and Inclusivity. Retrieved July 06, 2020, from https://www.dancespirit.com/10-black-ballerinas-carrying-on-misty-copelands-legacy-2530899384.html

Lewin, Y., & Collins, J. (2015). *Night's Dancer: The Life of Janet Collins*. Middletown, CT: Wesleyan University Press.

The Official Website of Misty Copeland. (n.d.). Retrieved July 06,

2020, from https://mistycopeland.com/

Stieg, C. (2018, February 5). 7 Iconic Black Women Who Changed the Course of Ballet History. Retrieved July 06, 2020, from https://www.refinery29.com/en-us/black-ballerinas-dancers-misty-copeland

DANCING WITH GAUCHOS

Peter Benjamin

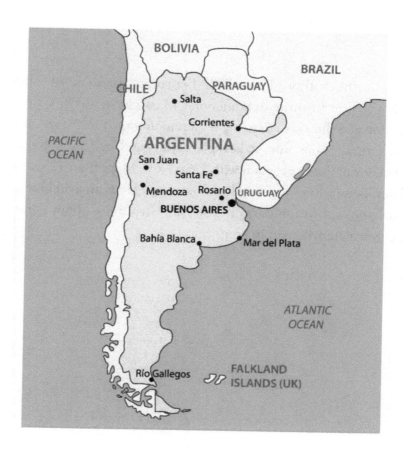

About the author: Peter Will Benjamin, founder of The Connection Institute in Somerville, Massachusetts, USA, first discovered the joy of dancing on a remote ranch in Patagonia, Argentina. This story takes place during Peter's year-long, transformational program with Leap Now. More than 12 years later, Peter's love of dance has flourished. He is an avid blues, bachata, and fusion dancer. You can learn more about Peter at www.peterwbenjamin.com.

Kilometer after kilometer slipped by as the Jeep sped along the snaking dirt road. I'd never felt as small as I did now, dwarfed by this epic landscape. Jagged mountains reached up toward a seemingly endless sky. The earth was dry and stark, its beauty contained in shades of brown, white, and tan, with pops of light green. Creeks and rivers were mostly hidden from sight, tucked into the region's many valleys.

Next to me, at the wheel, sat *El Patrón* (The Boss). El Patrón owned the 100,000-acre ranch in Argentina's Neuquén Province where I would be living for the next three months. His property was located in the northeastern Andes: the heart of Patagonia and the homeland of the gauchos.

I'd read about gauchos on the internet. Years ago, these *bolas*-wielding South American cowboys were utterly free. They roamed the vast plains of the Pampas, kept to themselves, and lived off the land.

While most gauchos work as animal handlers on ranches today, they've kept their mystique. They are skilled horsemen renowned for their ability to train horses to respond to soft touches, gentle coaxing, and whispers.

As I was choosing among various volunteer opportunities, the chance to spend time with these iconic figures became my deciding factor. I imagined working alongside them during the day and spending quiet evenings around the campfire.

I was deep in a daydream as we rumbled through a wrought iron gate. The entry sign read *Estancia Colipilli* (Colipilli Ranch). We had arrived.

A fellow volunteer named Cam showed me to my room. He was a lanky, young American whose friendliness instantly put me at ease.

"It's not much, but you'll get used to it," Cam told me as we approached a crumbling structure with whitewashed stone walls and a corrugated tin roof. Inside, there were two beds. Hanging between them were various goat parts, including a full rack of ribs that had been put up to dry. It smelled like you would imagine, and the meat was attracting flies. In that moment, reality hit: I was in a culture very different than any I had ever known.

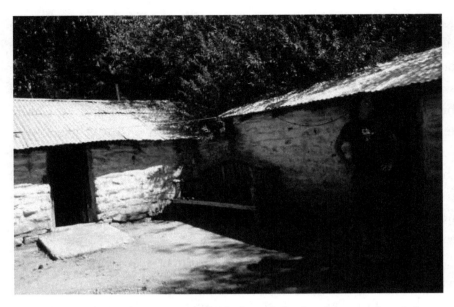

Cam, with the housing on the left and the kitchen on the right
Photo credit: Peter Will Benjamin

"I brought a tent," I told Cam. "I think I'll set that up."

Cam smiled understandingly.

"Yeah, it's different here," he said.

"When did you arrive?" I asked, ready to change the subject.

"Just a month ago," he replied. "I'm still new, but I speak Spanish. I'm happy to help you figure things out and to translate."

This was good news: my Spanish was tenuous at best.

Later that evening, I headed to the kitchen for dinner. The rickety wooden door opened to a room that was dark and filled with smoke from a wood-burning stove. In the center of the space, a big iron stake held the rack of ribs that had previously hung in my would-be bedroom. Through the haze, I saw I was not alone: Cam was there, as were four gauchos.

Each gaucho sat by himself. There in the dark room, they seemed as mysterious and solitary as I'd imagined them to be. It didn't seem like this was the time to introduce myself.

I approached Cam.

"What's for dinner?" I asked.

"Asado," Cam responded, handing me a knife. "Dinner around here is pretty casual. Go ahead and cut off a piece of meat for yourself."

I realized, then, that the dry, grizzled meat hanging in the center of the room would be my meal. I'd never seen anything like this, and I'd always been taught *not* to eat food that had been sitting out. With no other options, however, I tentatively approached the rack of ribs. Feeling slightly nauseated, I sliced off a hunk of the goat meat and took a bite.

The flavor was incredible: an explosion of umami. The outside of the meat was hard and crispy, while the inside was melt-in-your-mouth tender. I'd never had anything like it before, and have not had a better meal to this day.

"This is amazing!" I said to Cam. "How do they make it?"

"Asados are a goat leg or a rack of ribs," he told me. "They rinse the meat, rub it with salt, and cook it over coals for about two hours. The salt helps create an outside seal that allows the meat to roast in its own juices."

"Is this a traditional way of cooking?" I asked.

"It is!" Cam responded.

I would later learn that the gauchos had developed the technique. Back in the early days, a gaucho would slaughter a cow when he needed to eat. Since gauchos rode and lived alone, they couldn't possibly eat all of the meat before it spoiled; they needed to find a way to preserve it. When asado was first created, the Argentine people considered it unsanitary. Now, however, it's a popular traditional meal.

After dinner that night, Cam prepared me for the next day.

"Early tomorrow, we'll leave to begin work," he told me. "We'll be fixing fences and doing other manual labor, so dress accordingly. Also, pack a bag. We'll be gone for a few days."

The next morning, Cam was waiting for me with a piece of fresh, fried bread. As we sat together, eating our breakfast, one of the gauchos approached.

"Peter, this is Martín," Cam said, introducing us. "Martín, Pedro."

"Hola, Pedro!" Martín said, giving me a goofy, excited smile and a firm handshake.

Martín's hands were rough and calloused, as if he had worked hard every day of his life. I was surprised by what I perceived to be his dapper appearance, given that we were about to head off to do manual labor. Martín wore a button-up, collared shirt with its sleeves rolled up, topped with a hand-made wool vest. He also had on traditional gaucho pants known as *bombachas*, which have four lines of ruffles that run along both sides from the hip to the ankle. The bottom of the pants had a strap that ensured they were fastened tightly around Martín's ankles to prevent them from getting caught on anything while he rode.

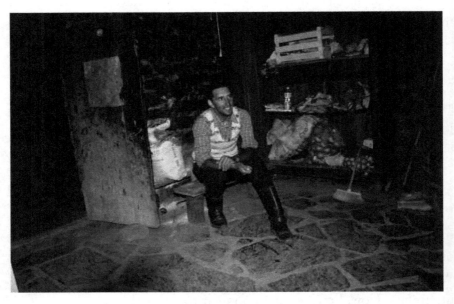

Martín in the kitchen of Estancia Colipilli
Photo credit: Peter Will Benjamin

Around his waist, Martín had fastened a red-and-black fabric belt called a *faja*, which was four inches wide and emblazoned with fantastic woven designs. It was a gallant-looking accessory that doubled as a way for Martín to hold his *facón*, a traditional gaucho knife.

"The plan for today is to ride three hours into the *campo* – that means 'countryside' – where we'll work for the next five days," Cam explained to me. "Because this property is so huge, we typically trek out to one area, do our work, and then come back."

Martín guided his horse and two others back toward us. As he came closer, I noticed there was something different about these animals: their manes were short! Martín must have noticed me staring, because he said something in Spanish.

"He's saying that he crops the horse's hair, just like he crops his own," Cam translated. Martín ran his fingers through his own short hair and then said something that made Cam chortle.

"He said you can tell the gringo horses because they look like hippies," Cam said. Seeing my smile, Martín let out a dorky laugh.

"He also does it to keep burrs out of their manes," Cam added.

We saddled up and began our journey into the countryside. As we traveled, I became lost in thought. I'd never been this far from a city. Where I'd grown up, just outside Boston, everything had been nearby: grocery stores, my friends, and entertainment. To arrive here, however, I'd flown to Buenos Aires, spent 18 hours on a bus, and traveled six hours with El Patrón. The nearest town was a three-hour journey on horseback from Estancia Colipilli, and I was currently heading in the opposite direction. I was in a remote corner of Argentina, riding a horse alongside a gaucho. I breathed deeply, contentedly. The countryside smelled of dry earth and grass.

After a few more hours, we arrived at our campsite. There, a lone tree stood with a large tarp draped over one of the branches. I saw a deep hole in the ground, which Cam explained would keep our campfires safe from the wind. Nearby, there was a creek where we could gather water. In the distance, mountains painted with shrubs and bushes loomed beneath the massive azure sky.

Today was not a day to work. It was a day to arrive, set up camp, and settle in. I unrolled my sleeping bag and set about making a fire. It was crackling in no time, and Martín got out ingredients to make our dinner. We would be making *tortas fritas* (fried bread) from scratch using animal fat, oil, salt, flour, and yeast.

That evening, as we prepared our simple meal, Martín told us about the first gauchos.

"They were people of the land," he said as he sprinkled yeast into a depression in the pile of flour. "They had very few belongings: just their horses and things they made themselves."

Martín began to knead warm water mixed with oil and salt into the mixture to make the dough.

"Because the gauchos knew how to survive, the government eventually drafted many of them into the army. They fought in *el Guerra del desierto* (the Desert War) and many others. That was when we began using facones."

He paused for a moment.

"Now we wait for the yeast to activate," he announced as he sat back and looked out at the mountains.

"What happened after the wars?" Cam asked.

"The gauchos went back to the countryside. They hadn't been working, so they had no money, and few of them remembered how to live off the land. That's why we began working for the estancias. Now, we build and fix fences, tend horses, and help manage cattle. None of us lives like the first gauchos did, but it's my dream to one day buy my own land and to survive off what I can grow, raise, and make."

We sat in silence for a while until Martín signaled that the tortas were ready to fry. He showed us how to tear off pieces of dough in a twisting motion, ball them up, and then pinch them into a flat circle.

"The fat can't be too hot, or the tortas won't cook evenly," he told us as he dropped a perfect disc onto the frying pan. We ate the tortas fritas in batches as they came out of the pan, continuing until all the dough was used up and our bellies were full.

That night, I slept beneath the open sky, admiring unfamiliar stars. In the Southern Hemisphere, constellations like Orion's Belt were replaced by some I'd never seen, such as the Southern Cross. The stars shone brilliantly: in this arid region, clouds rarely obstructed the view.

The night noises I'd known in Boston, like the chirp of crickets or the buzz of mosquitos, were notably absent. The wind through the grass and the occasional whinny of a horse were the only interruption of the quiet.

***

"*Arriba*, Pedro." Martín said gently, almost singing. "*Es la manana.*" (Get up, Peter; it's morning.) I opened my eyes. The stars were still out, and there was only a hint of sunlight on the horizon.

"Will you make the fire?" Martín asked me.

I got out of my sleeping bag and stumbled about for a bit, gathering kindling. All the wood was dry, so I was able to light a nice little fire in short order. We made *maté*, the caffeinated tea the gauchos liked to drink each morning, and Cam and I ate a few tortas.

After this basic breakfast, we saddled up the horses and headed out to the fence line. We spent our morning digging post holes, replacing wire, re-securing old posts, and switching others out. About lunchtime, we headed back to the camp to eat and take a *siesta* (nap). Then, there was more work until dinnertime.

This became our routine. Each day, we fixed fences across the wide expanse of the Patagonian pampas. Each night, we would build a fire, make dinner, and sit together in the pristine stillness.

At the end of that week, we returned to Estancia Colipilli. While I had thought of this homebase as quite basic before, it now seemed to be a place of abundance. There were one or two others we could talk with in the evenings; we could light a fire in the furnace and wash our clothes, and our meals became slightly more versatile with the occasional addition of tomato sauce—a special treat that people would sometimes bring us when they had visited a town.

Martín's girlfriend also came to visit him that Sunday afternoon.

"How often does he get to see her?" I asked Cam.

"About once a month," he told me. "It's that way with all the gauchos I have met. One gaucho here is married, and his wife lives in town. He's retired, so he could go and be with her, but he prefers to live out here."

I don't think I could do that, I thought. *The gauchos really do like to be alone.*

The weeks went by. Martín, Cam, and I spent Monday through Friday mending fences on the pampas and our weekends at Estancia Colipilli. As autumn deepened, the mountains burst into color, bringing new hues of bright red, yellow, and orange to the landscape.

Around this time, El Patrón announced that volunteers would begin lodging in Estancia Ranquilco, the main ranch house. It was the only winterized structure on his property, and he wanted us to be comfortable as the weather turned colder.

Estancia Ranquilco was a few hours away on horseback, or a day's walk. With nothing else to do, I packed my belongings into my backpack and set off on foot. Around mid-afternoon, I saw Estancia Ranquilco in the distance. The home was beautiful, made of locally sourced lumber and surrounded by peach trees. It stood out against the backdrop of the Andes Mountains and the rushing Trocoman River.

I was met at the door by an older woman, who introduced herself as the house manager.

"I'll show you to your room," she said, leading me down a small path past an overgrown garden and a chicken house to a humble but sturdy cabin. "Make sure to come over to the main house after you're settled in. It's one of the volunteer's birthdays today, so we're doing something special."

I could smell amazing aromas wafting from the kitchen. Hungry from my trek, and excited to see what was in store, I unpacked quickly and went to find the others. I eventually located them outside the back door on an open-air, tiled patio.

Cam was there, along with the house manager, a few Argentine women, some volunteers, and a young woman I recognized from a few of her visits to Estancia Colipilli. She was El Patrón's daughter, Skye, whom Cam and I called *La Gaucha*. We had nicknamed as many things as we could: star clusters, mountains that caught our fancy, and the resident animals. It helped bring a sense of the personal and familiar to a world that was so different from what we'd previously known.

Skye had been raised living half of each year in the United States and half at El Ranquilco, so she was familiar with both cultures. She spoke English and Spanish fluently, rode a horse like an expert, and was one tough woman. At some point, a horse had kicked her leg, causing part of her muscle to tear and roll up. Now it was a bulge just below the side of her knee. I imagined that had hurt like hell, but she had never gone to see a doctor.

Skye's boyfriend was a gaucho. He and four other gauchos – more than I'd ever seen together before – were also there. Per usual, they were dressed impeccably, wearing leather jerkin pants and button-down shirts.

Initially, seeing everyone made me uncomfortable. This was the largest number of people I'd been around since arriving at the ranch. My discomfort faded into delight as one of the volunteers handed me a freshly prepared empanada. I'd eaten little besides goat, potatoes, onions, and rice for the last three months, so the flaky crust felt like a decadent treat.

Martín, who was talking with some of the other gauchos, called me over. He helped me into a vest made from brown-and-cream cowhide. I understood that he was loaning it to me as something special to wear on this festive occasion.

Not a minute after I'd put on the vest, Skye's boyfriend began to play his guitar. His gaze focused inward, he smiled gently as his music became the backdrop to our gathering. He strummed softly at first, until the wistful music inspired one couple to begin to dance slowly together.

"What is this music?" I asked Skye.

"He's playing different types of traditional folk songs," she replied.

The energy built organically from there. The gaucho, now dividing his attention between his playing and the dancing, sat up a little straighter. The next song he played was more lively and drew another couple into the center of the stone patio. The music's tempo was now moderato, and the dancers were starting to grab everyone's attention. What had been background music became the focus of our group experience.

Before I knew it, the music had ticked up to a more lively pace. The guitar player was now watching the dancers intently. When he finished the next song, rather than beginning a new tune, he pulled out a little boombox and some cassette tapes. As soon as he hit "play," the energy changed again.

What came on must have been a popular song, since all the gauchos and several of the women stood up to dance. They smiled, whooped, and exuded more joy than I'd seen from anyone since I'd arrived. Even gentle, reserved Martín was letting loose.

I watched as the gauchos and their partners clapped, stepped, and stomped along to the music. I wanted to join in, but my shyness held me back. I had never seen people dance together like this before – with such joy and abandon – and I had certainly never danced myself.

Luckily, because of the lack of available partners, Skye soon pulled me from my seat. In keeping with her strong, decisive nature, she began to lead, teaching me the moves as we did them.

"This dance is called the *corrido*, or 'the run,'" she told me. "Bend your knees and feel the pulse of the music."

She held my right hand in her left, and wrapped her other arm around my waist. I tried to relax as she guided me through the steps.

Eventually I began dancing competently enough that Skye allowed me to lead. I loved the feeling of moving to the music with another person, and I felt a little starstruck to be partnered with La Gaucha.

When the song ended, I sat down, exhilarated.

Next, I decided to watch Skye and her boyfriend dance. As the music began again, they moved together, so in sync that they resembled one living organism. I was astounded, never having seen partner dancing before. As I looked on, I had no idea that partner dancing would become one of the central parts of my life two years later.

Next, the ladies took over the boombox. Looking through the available cassettes, they pulled out a few tapes and began to DJ. As they played different types of music, I learned more dance styles.

I got a crash course in *chamamé*, a couples' dance from northeastern Argentina done in closed embrace to upbeat music. The atmosphere at our little party became more lively as couples stepped across the floor to the sounds of Spanish guitar and accordions. Learning corrido had been a good warmup. La Gaucha was once again my teacher, and I was reminded of how strong she was. I swooned a little as she guided me.

Next, there was *ranchera*, which is a partner dance that looks similar to a waltz.

The name comes from the word *ranchos*, since the songs originated on ranches in rural Mexico. As this dance was more complicated than the others, I took a seat and helped myself to more empanadas.

Before long, we were back to more beginner-friendly styles: *cumbia* and *merengue*. I enjoyed cumbia, a dance from Colombia, but merengue was perplexing to me. I watched, confused, as one of the young women began moving her hips to the music in a way that looked unnatural: her torso stayed relatively still, while her hips swung side to side to the beat of the music. I didn't appreciate the way it looked, which is amusing to me now. I would learn years later that this is the proper way to do it, and that the young woman was a better merengue dancer than everyone else there that night. Now that I've taken classes, I like moving my hips that way, too.

As the night wore on, we moved from dancing every song, to dancing occasionally, to simply sitting together talking on the patio. Eventually, someone turned off the boombox. Skye's boyfriend picked up his guitar again and began to play slow, soulful ballads as the sun set behind the Andes.

Within half an hour, the only light left was from lanterns on the porch and the starry sky above. In the profound silence of the Patagonian night, the gaucho's music was a pure, crystalline sound, floating into the expanse of the countryside.

In between songs, we feasted on asado, empanadas, and freshly picked peaches that had been warmed by the afternoon sun. After so much time alone in the middle of nowhere, with so few options for what to do or eat, this was ecstasy. The merriment, flavors, and social interaction were made sweeter by their rarity. We savored each moment, knowing not to take anything for granted.

That night, I had a special glimpse into the world of the gauchos. Despite all my reading about their culture, I never could have imagined a moment like this: a time when these typically isolated men laughed, danced, and delighted in their broken solitude.

Recommended resources:

Neuquén Province. (2020, July 01). Retrieved July 08, 2020, from https://en.wikipedia.org/wiki/Neuqu%C3%A9n_Province

Sessa, A. (2018). *Gauchos: Icons of Argentina*. New York, NY: Assouline.

Waring, R. (2009). *The Gauchos of Argentina*. Boston, MA: Heinle/Cengage Learning.

THE ACCIDENTAL AUDITION

Laurie Bonner-Baker

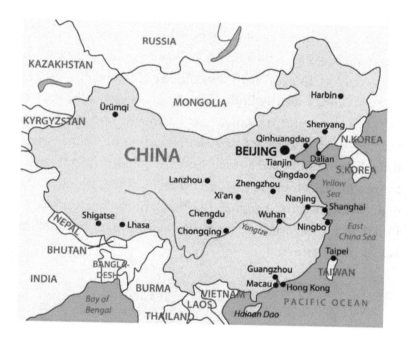

About the author: Laurie is a music teacher, musician, and lindy hopper who currently works at an international school in Kuala Lumpur. Laurie began lindy hopping in 2003 through classes at Willowbrook Ballroom in Chicago and the University of Illinois Swing Society in Champaign-Urbana, Illinois. Since learning lindy hop, she has been lucky enough to travel the world dancing, making music, and teaching at international schools across Asia, including in China, where the following story takes place. Some highlights from Laurie's travels in Asia include giving classes in collegiate shag at a dance workshop in Shanghai, playing baritone saxophone in a funk band in Beijing, and attending various dance workshops across the continent.

When I left my house in Beijing on Saturday morning, I intended to go to dance practice for a couple of hours. When I returned home, well after dark, I had auditioned for a Hollywood movie.

To understand how this adventure unfolded, you need to know a few things. First off, I had been living in Beijing for less than a month. Having just taken a job at an international school, I was still settling in. The year was 2013, and many of the technologies we know today – such as translation and rideshare apps – were not available. Furthermore, the Great Chinese Firewall and my lack of a good Chinese SIM card blocked my access to a lot of information. Because of this, as well as my extremely limited Mandarin language skills, I was primed for the sort of miscommunication that led to my accidental audition.

Not long after my arrival in Beijing, I realized I'd taken many things for granted in the United States. In my hometown of Chicago, for instance, I could go dancing with relative ease. I would take the train, my car, or my bike and be at my local swing dance venue within 20 minutes. Going out in Beijing, however, was a different story.

Before leaving my house, I would write the name of my destination in Mandarin on a small notecard. I would then head outside and try to catch a taxi. This was before the days of Uber (or Didi or Grab), and taxis in my suburban neighborhood were uncommon. Thus, I was gambling on three accounts: 1) that there would be a taxi; 2) that I'd written the Mandarin characters correctly and the driver would be able to read my handwriting; and 3) that he would know the location of the dance venue. A driver's knowledge was the only form of GPS available then.

My notecard method worked three quarters of the time. When it didn't, I would climb out of the taxi and wait in the acrid-smelling, polluted air for another. At some point, I would finally be on my way to the dance venue: an old building located on a pedestrian-only street in the Russian district of the city.

I loved this place. Like many people from Chicago, I have Polish ancestry, and the smell of sauerkraut and other Eastern European foods reminded me of my childhood. Passing by Russian bakeries, grocery stores, and restaurants, I felt right at home. My appreciation for the area was further deepened by its charming quirks. One of the local stores had a pet pig that always stayed out front and wandered as far as his leash would allow. The people-watching was also fantastic. At night, patrons of a tacky nearby nightclub were everywhere, and they were all dressed like characters from *Night at the Roxbury*.

I always looked forward to my jaunt down this street, not just because of the scenery, but also because of the excitement I felt before the event. As you might imagine, moving to a new country by yourself can be lonely, and dancing was one of the things that helped Beijing feel more like home.

As I neared the lindy hop venue, I could barely keep from skipping. I couldn't wait to get onto the dance floor!

The lindy hop community in Beijing welcomed me with open arms. In my first few visits to the venue, everyone asked me to dance, and I met many new people. Having traveled extensively, I was familiar with the warmth of swing communities around the world, and counted on it when I arrived in a new location. I knew that Beijing's scene had started in 2003, when an American of Chinese descent named Adam had begun offering classes at a local venue called the CD Jazz Cafe. While Adam had initially received most interest from expats, by 2013 the lindy hop community in Beijing was beginning to attract more locals, some of whom were helping run the events. Coincidentally, Adam had returned to the United States to pursue a master's degree in music education just before my arrival.

My new acquaintances included members of Beijing's swing performance team, who came from many different backgrounds. There was a woman named Leru from Russia who had trained and taught extensively with Adam, and who seemed to be one of the most experienced dancers in the scene. There was also Zeng, a talented Chinese dancer who was one of Adam's former students. Zeng was teaching, helping organize the performance team, and leading efforts to recruit more local dancers into the lindy hop community.

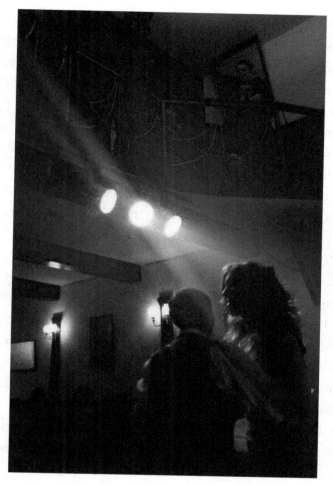

The author dances balboa, another dance of the swing era, with a friend at a venue called Modernista in Beijing in November 2013
Photo credit: Anonymous

I also met other Chinese nationals on the team, including George, whom I spoke with in English since he had studied abroad in the United States, and a friendly, outgoing woman named Miranda. There were more expats, too: Josh, an American from New York who helped run the scene, Richard, an older German man, and many others.

Those who spoke English told me more about the team. There were various ethnicities of Chinese dancers represented, they said, and people danced at different levels. The more experienced dancers were helping to train up new talent.

Leru was, indeed, the most experienced dancer in Beijing then, having danced lindy hop for more than 15 years. Her movement, honed over countless hours of practice, was refined and dynamic. At the time, Leru was a prominent organizer in Swing Beijing, the first and only company in the city to teach classes and run events based on swing-era dances. In addition to teaching lindy hop and balboa, I learned, she also taught burlesque classes and organized a burlesque troupe.

After a few conversations, when the dancers learned I had been on a performance team in Chicago, they invited me to join their next rehearsal. I eagerly accepted, excited for the chance to make new friends and nostalgic for my team back home.

A few days later, dressed in purple, zebra-pattern exercise leggings and a neon yellow workout top, I arrived at the studio (late, since the taxi driver had gotten lost) ready to practice. The group was already hard at work, with several couples running through a high-energy routine. From the emails I'd received, I knew they had been working on this routine for some kind of audition, but I wasn't sure when the audition was, or what it was for.

Several of the dancers who had been watching the rehearsal got up to greet me. They didn't speak English, but it didn't matter; they led me to a corner of the room and began to show me the moves from the choreography. I was just catching on when everybody began to pack up their things.

What in the world is going on? I wondered. Practice just started.

As I looked around, some of the team members seemed to be giving directions to others. Since everything was happening in Mandarin, however, I wasn't sure what they were saying. A hurried energy swept through the room as everyone moved toward the door. Over the next few minutes, my attempts to figure out what was happening all fell flat. Each time I approached George, Josh, Leru, or one of the other English speakers, they would be pulled away by someone else. It was a bit of a frenzy.

Finally, when we'd left the studio and were halfway down the stairwell, Zeng approached me.

"We're on our way to an audition," he said. "The bus is here, and we need to go. Come on!"

This was all I got before he disappeared. And while I still had no specifics as to what the audition was for or where exactly we were headed, I decided to go along. I had no other plans for the day, and I thought it would be fun to watch the team perform.

"It's great you're coming!" Leru said to me as I boarded the private, air-conditioned bus waiting in front of the building. "Since you're an advanced dancer, we might use you to demonstrate some lindy hop."

I shrugged off her comment. This wasn't *my* audition, after all. As I took my seat, I wondered if anyone had meant to tell me about this excursion. Perhaps they thought I could read the Mandarin in the group's text chain, or maybe the person charged with sharing information with me had forgotten. I couldn't be sure.

As the bus headed out of the city and into the countryside, the dancers taught me new words in Mandarin. I also had a chance to chat with the other English speakers about our lives and Chinese history. However, when I pressed for more details about the day – such as where this private bus had come from, how long we would be staying at our destination, or what the audition was for – I received vague answers.

Within an hour, the scenery had changed from tall, grey buildings to open fields. The air, no longer heavy with city pollution, became sweet with the scent of grass and flowers. Because of this idyllic, bucolic setting, I was surprised by what appeared a few minutes later: a massive compound made up of large concrete buildings that resembled airline hangars.

"That's the movie lot!" George said.

"The audition is for a movie?" I asked, wondering why this information had been so hard to get before this moment.

"Yes!" he replied. "We are meeting the film's choreographer today. He's the one who sent the bus!"

As we disembarked, we were met by a fast-talking Chinese receptionist who ushered us inside one of the nearby buildings. The interior was as gorgeous as the outside was plain. There were high ceilings and marble-floored hallways full of gold accents. The receptionist led us to bathrooms where she said we could change.

I followed the other ladies into the women's room, where they all began to get ready, applying stage makeup and putting on black skirts and white blouses. They twirled their hair into 1940s-style victory rolls, spritzing their new 'dos liberally with hairspray and accessorizing them with brightly colored, clip-in flowers.

It only got fancier from there. Leru pulled on a sequin-laden flapper dress and matching heels. She topped off her look with a black, bobbed wig held firmly in place by multitudes of bobby pins.

I stood there, watching this transformation in surprised silence. These women looked fantastic and elegant, and I looked like the exercise instructor from a 1980s workout video.

"Maybe this is okay," I thought. "I'm just here to watch."

Exiting the bathroom, we met up with the leads, who were now dressed in suits and bow ties. They were waiting with a middle-aged Black American man who greeted us in English. Although he was dressed casually, I knew immediately that he was the choreographer. He stood tall, radiated confidence, and emitted a laid-back professional vibe. While he was friendly, something about him also felt tired, as if he'd been out of LA and in the Chinese countryside for a little longer than he'd have liked.

"It's great to meet you," he said flatly. "My team and I are excited to see what you've put together."

I sheepishly hung toward the back of the group as the choreographer led us into a huge rehearsal space with beautiful hardwood floors. At the front of the room sat his crew of ridiculously attractive, Los Angeles-based counterparts. Each person was young, trim, and well dressed. I felt like I was meeting the cast of *Black Swan*.

At first, I was excited to see that the dancers were American. It had been almost a month since I'd been around a group of people who shared my culture. A minute later, however, the reality sank in: these were real professionals with formal training, very unlike our group of rag-tag, hobbyist lindy hoppers. I wondered apprehensively how the team's performance would be received.

Nonetheless, the team stayed confident. They ran their routine for the panel, who looked on solemnly and clapped politely afterward.

"Now," the choreographer said standing up. "We'd like to see some lindy hop social dancing."

"Laurie, we need you for this," Leru said.

"Excuse me?" I replied, surprised.

"Yes!" she insisted. "You're one of the more experienced social dancers in the group. This is why we wanted you to come along."

I really must have missed that memo, I thought, as my heart started to race.

I made my way to the front of the group, my garish neon purple and yellow outfit a stark contrast to the glamorous black-and-white clothes of my fellow performers. Standing there, I wasn't sure whether to be mortified or thrilled. I was intimidated by the idea of dancing in front of any audience, let alone this group of professional dancers. But apparently, I was auditioning for a movie!

Because I am tall, one of the team members paired me with the tallest lead, who looked as startled by this decision as I felt. I'd danced at least once with the other leads at the weekly social, but never with him. As we were unfamiliar with one another's styles, this match was not ideal. Despite my concerns, I went with it.

"Show us your best moves!" the choreographer instructed us as he turned on a song.

We formed a semicircle and began clapping to the beat as each couple took turns dancing in the center. The more experienced performers did aerials, flips, and other fancy moves. They looked great in their matching outfits, moving with the precision and confidence of long-time partners.

My lead and I had no moves to speak of. After a few awkward moments communicating via my broken Mandarin and hand gestures, I was pretty sure we had decided to stick to the basics. I mustered all my enthusiasm in order to make the most of our simple performance. As we entered the jam circle, I hoped my amped-up energy, massive smile, and zebra tights would at least be memorable. While it wouldn't be my best performance, I was happy to support the team in the social dancing part of this tryout.

At the end of the song, after all the couples had had their moment to shine, the choreographer stood up. I was feeling high off the energy of performance, and also relieved that my part of the audition was over.

"Now we want to see some solo moves from each of you," the choreographer said. "Starting from stage left, you'll dance across the floor, stop in the middle for your spotlight performance, and then dance your way off."

Each of you, I realized, meant me, too.

My stomach dropped as the jazz classic "Sing, Sing, Sing" began to play. While I felt confident in my partner work, I was terrible at dancing alone. I didn't practice solo movement, and I had never before taken classes in solo Charleston, Big Apple, or other, similar jazz styles and choreographies. I'd never felt my lanky body looked good doing this part of the art form, so I'd never worked on building my skills. To make matters worse, the song was *fast*.

Feeling awkward, I waited in line and watched as my new teammates started dancing across the room. I was growing more nervous with each passing second. When it was finally my turn, I danced my gangly heart out in front of that panel of unreasonably good-looking professional dancers. While I wish I could tell you more about this part of the experience, I have very few memories of it. I imagine my brain blocked them out to keep me from feeling mortified later on.

Despite all our best efforts, I could tell the panel was unimpressed. They sat at their table and watched, politely nodding as each person performed. Luckily, sequin-laden Leru was the last to go. She sashayed her way across the floor, showing off with high kicks and swivels. The panel looked delighted (or perhaps relieved) to see her talent. She struck a pose as the song ended, her sequins sparkling under the lights as she held her position in the center of the room.

"You're the star!" the choreographer burst out, clapping his hands for Leru. "Thank you for such a bangin' audition."

He motioned for all of us to come closer.

"We'll let you know about the film in a couple of weeks," he said. "Before you head home, please go enjoy a free dinner at our restaurant. We want to thank you for coming all the way out here."

After all the travel and dancing, we were hungry, and eagerly accepted the offer.

The on-site restaurant was just as fancy as the audition space. A waiter led us to an ornately carved, dark wooden table surrounded by traditional paintings, where he invited us to sit down on plush chairs. At the center of the table was a gigantic lazy Susan, which is used in traditional Chinese meals.

There were no menus. Instead, the chef brought out course after course of freshly prepared dishes. There was Peking duck, a tasty dumpling soup, loads of noodles, a whole cooked fish, and bowls and bowls of fluffy rice. We washed it all down with Tsingtao, a tasty, popular beer made at China's second-largest brewery.

A few hours later, stuffed with the most delicious dinner I'd had since arriving in Beijing, we made our way back to the bus. We climbed aboard quietly, everyone tired from the busy day and massive meal. As we pulled out of the parking lot, we rolled down the windows. The smell of summer was on the evening breeze. It was a refreshing break from Beijing's smoggy city air, and reminded me of nights in Chicago.

I took a deep breath as I thought more about the day's whirlwind events. I imagined my zebra tights and questionable solo performance would not merit me a spot in the film, but it didn't matter. I was full of gratitude for this spontaneous, random adventure that would serve as a foundation for new friendships.

Over my next four years in China, these relationships would grow. In particular, I would learn many things from Leru, who would teach me not only how to move, pose, and perform with confidence and grace, but also how to be a strong, savvy business woman. The accidental audition, combined with my ensuing experiences, confirmed what I've learned as I've danced my way through every transition in life: while you can never guess where dancing abroad will take you, it's safe to say that it will lead to memorable adventures.

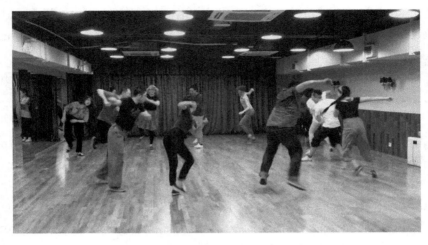

Laurie rehearses the Big Apple routine with the
Beijing performance team in the spring of 2017
Photo credit: Anonymous

Recommended resources:

Frankie Manning Ambassador Program. (2020). Retrieved July 07, 2020, from https://www.frankiemanningfoundation.org/ambassador-program/

Manning, F., & Millman, C. R. (2008). *Frankie Manning: Ambassador of Lindy Hop*. Philadelphia, PA, PA: Temple Univ. Press.

Miller, N., & Jensen, E. (1996). *Swingin' at the Savoy: The Memoir of a Jazz Dancer*. Philadelphia, PA: Temple University Press.

Swing Beijing. (n.d.). Retrieved July 07, 2020, from https://swingbeijing.com/

Swift, R. (2019, July 23). The Track 041 - Sing Lim. Retrieved July 07, 2020, from http://www.thetrackpodcast.com/episodes/041

PART 4: PERSONAL DEVELOPMENT

*"Dance enables you to find yourself and lose
yourself at the same time."*
—Anonymous

As a life coach, supporting this section's authors was doubly fulfilling for me. Not only did we get to geek out about story arcs and character development, but we also dove deeply into the ways in which dance challenges us to grow.

These stories capture the highs and lows inherent in personal development work. As we go through the self-exploration process, we may be surprised, confronted, disappointed, or even disgusted as we discover the conditioned beliefs and habits that influence our lives.

This work is well worth the effort. As you'll see, dance provides these authors with a way to reflect on who they are and to become a better version of themselves. Through movement, they heal old wounds, release limiting beliefs, shed behaviors that hold them back, and explore meaningful parts of their identity.

I AM HERE

Khalila Fordham

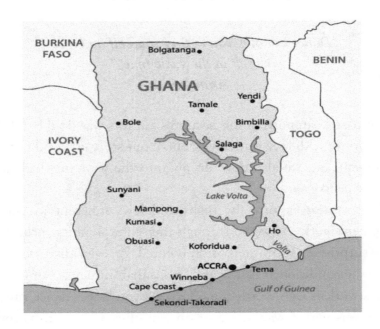

About the author: Khalila Fordham, PsyD, is a lifelong dancer, as well as the multicultural support specialist and a staff psychologist at the University of Puget Sound in Tacoma, Washington, USA.

In addition to conducting therapy, Khalila has an affinity for social justice and public education. She advocates for and mentors youth who are underrepresented and experience risk factors. Khalila has organized and facilitated community outreach programs on mental health, stress management, sex education, sexual assault prevention, team building, and prejudice and discrimination reduction.

Khalila is working toward her certification as an AASECT sex therapist, specializing in trauma recovery, taboo lifestyle practices, and treatment of individuals from marginalized identity groups. She also recently stepped into the foray of entrepreneurship by co-founding Anomalous Partners, a company dedicated to developing and disseminating resources for positive change in society. The firm is preparing to launch its first podcast in the upcoming months.

In her free time, Khalila enjoys reading, dancing, singing, playing the violin, practicing Brazilian jiu jitsu, attending sci-fi conventions, and engaging in intense discussions. She also is a member of Delta Sigma Theta Sorority, Incorporated.

"*Que linda!*" ("How beautiful!") said a man emphatically as I walked by him. It was 9 p.m. on a summer night in Buenos Aires, and I was coming home from my first tango class. I had been daydreaming about nights at *milongas* (tango dance halls) in the city when the man's words pulled me from my reverie and from my reverie and into the present moment on this dark street.

"*De dónde sos?*" ("Where are you from?") the man next to him asked longingly, as he grabbed my hand and attempted to pull me closer.

My eyes widened in surprise at their forwardness. I pulled my hand back, turned away, and quickened my pace, hoping to return to my residence before anything else happened.

It was my third year of college, and I'd chosen to study abroad in Buenos Aires, intending to hone my Spanish skills and explore the world of tango. While my experiences in the country had been incredible so far, I'd noticed that I was receiving far more attention from men than my white classmates were. So, after several incidents within the first few days, I approached my program coordinator.

"Lots of guys are catcalling me and even grabbing me," I said. "Do you know why that might be?"

She paused for a moment and then hesitantly began to tell me about the history of slavery in Argentina, as well as the subsequent genocide of Black people in the country.

"After most of the Black population was killed, many of the remaining Black women either married white men or were subjected to sex work for survival," she said. "Unfortunately, this created a stereotype that dark-skinned women are promiscuous."

I was shocked and disgusted. Why hadn't anyone told me about this before I arrived? In a new country for the first time, I was already outside of my comfort zone. Now, I was also afraid of what might happen to me based on the way I was perceived. I could have never guessed that the stereotypes of enslaved people would follow me here.

Since none of my classmates wanted to take tango classes with me, I stopped going. I didn't have money for taxis, and I didn't want to walk alone at night anymore. I was massively disappointed, as tango was one of the primary reasons I'd chosen to study abroad in Argentina.

Unfortunately, this experience was not foreign to me. It was not the first time my identity had impacted my life or my dancing, and it would not be the last.

***

For those who do not know, many Black Americans see the opportunity to dance as a gift to be honored. It's a way we celebrate life and express joy, as well as all other emotions. When we're dancing outside of Black or Brown communities, however, we often feel the need to censor ourselves for fear of being judged, sexualized, or persecuted for engaging in any behavior that differs from that of the majority group. In this way, dance is a sort of symbol for the rest of our lives.

My love of this art form first developed in the Black community in Atlanta, where I lived for some time. When I think about my childhood, I imagine that I moved in the pure, uninhibited way children can. I loved dance so much that, before I turned five, I wanted nothing more than to be a professional dancer. I adored the combination of agility, flexibility, poise, and grace I saw performers exuded on stage. As I got older, however, I began to feel an overwhelming sense of anxiety when I danced, especially in public. This was odd for me, as a typically vivacious, goofy young woman, and I attribute the shift in my behavior to many experiences of being marginalized, "othered," and at times actively discriminated against because of my skin color. While this happened many times, a few pivotal moments stand out to me.

One year, during my high school dance team's spring routine, each performer was given the liberty to freestyle during the first eight counts of the music. Some of my teammates and I decided to show the audience a few moves that highlighted our flexibility, and I even did the splits. The next day in class, one of the senior basketball players approached me.

"You would make a really good stripper," he told me.

"What?" I asked.

"You would make a really good stripper," he repeated. "I saw you doing those splits."

"Wait, so let me get this straight," I said, incredulously. "You think I should be a stripper just because I'm flexible? That's probably the dumbest thing I've ever heard."

While I wanted to pretend that the comment hadn't bothered me, I spent a lot of time afterward thinking about how people perceived the way that I move. It especially hurt that the young man hadn't commented on the white dancers' performance, despite having watched similar movements made by other members of the team. In that moment, I felt inappropriately sexualized, and as if all my creative choices had to be second-guessed. While I'd known that Black women in the United States are often hypersexualized as an ongoing consequence of slavery and oppression, this encounter made me realize I was not an exception to this phenomenon.

Moving forward, I became extremely vigilant about how I presented myself in public, and began to consciously and unconsciously present an adjusted persona whenever I was in the company of people of more than one race. I did whatever I could to be perceived as well educated and ladylike, including assuming the perfect posture I'd developed through years of training as a violinist, monitoring my language, and subduing my quirks to ensure that those around me would acknowledge my intelligence. It felt as if I were always hiding, strategically revealing as much as I felt comfortable to show, but never giving myself permission to be completely present.

My challenges with dance and true self-expression in general didn't end when I graduated from high school. As I went on to minor in dance in college, I became self-conscious that my body didn't resemble those glorified in the world of ballet. I'd noticed time and time again that most teachers preferred the thin, tall, white appearance for ballerinas and assumed that people who looked like that would dance best. I was lean and muscular, on the shorter side, and I had a slightly curvier body than what was considered ideal.

When practicing a new sequence in class or at an audition, I felt afraid to make mistakes. This was not just because ballet stresses perfection in technique, but because my skin color made me stand out from the rest of my classmates. I therefore worried that errors I made would be glaringly obvious, and that any mistakes would confirm assumptions that Black dancers lack ballet potential. For these reasons, I began to hide on the sidelines to avoid bringing attention to myself, even if this meant that I was not practicing enough to improve. Therefore, I never gave myself the opportunity to explore my full potential.

Over the ensuing years, dance became my hobby rather than my career. I continued on with my life, performing when I could, and starting work as a psychologist at the University of Puget Sound. That was where I met my colleague, and now friend, Professor LaToya Brackett.

In the spring of 2019, I learned Professor Brackett would be teaching a course that combined didactic learning on campus with an opportunity to study abroad in Ghana. I jumped at the chance to audit the course, as I was interested in studying more about the African Diaspora – the term commonly used to describe the mass dispersion of peoples from Africa during the Atlantic slave trade – and the subsequent disenfranchisement of the Black community in the United States. I also could not pass up the prospect of visiting my ancestral homeland. Thus, in December 2019, after the classroom portion of our course, I left the United States to travel to Accra, Ghana, where I would spend the next three weeks.

***

On our first full day in the country, to my surprise and delight, we had the privilege of attending a drumming and dance class at the University of Ghana, Accra. As I walked into the classroom, I relished that our teachers were Black. Most of my instructors in the United States, as well as my tango teacher in Argentina, had been white. Thus, whether I was taking ballet, jazz, hip hop, or tango, I was often one of the only Black people in the room, if not *the* only one.

Up until now, the dance experiences I'd had with other Black people had all come through my intentional effort, such as signing up for community classes with prominent Black artists or enrolling in extracurricular activities like my high school step team and college dance ensemble, in which my Black instructors were also my peers. I had never walked into a class and been surprised to find a Black teacher. Dancing in Ghana, I was discovering, would be vastly different than my experience dancing in Argentina and in the United States.

The lead instructor began the class by giving us some context.

"In West African countries, traditional drumming and dancing almost always go together," he said. "Connecting with the music makes you a better dancer, and vice versa. That's why we'll do both today."

An unfortunate consequence of having had so few Black teachers, particularly when learning dance styles that had originated within Black cultures, was that I had rarely, if ever, been provided with the full historical context of the arts I was learning. Thus, rather than feeling connected to the story within the dances, I'd just learned the moves and counts I needed to get right. As the instructor told us more about how drumming and dance here in Ghana are a part of communication and community building, I felt deeply grateful for this chance to connect with the meaning of these culturally rich art forms.

We would start by learning the music, he told us, inviting everyone to sit in a large circle with the drummers. These musicians then demonstrated a relatively simple sequence of three beats: *Ba dum bum. Ba dum bum. Ba dum bum.*

While it was fun to play, the meaning of the sequence resonated even more.

"Each beat of this rhythm represents a different word of a powerful phrase," our teacher said. "I. Am. Here."

He walked around the room as we hit the drums.

"Play assertively!" he told me. "Present yourself fully! Demand that you be acknowledged by announcing, 'I am here,' with your rhythm!"

Unsatisfied with our attempts, he began to work with people individually.

"Where are you?" he asked, attempting to ground each student in the present.

When one of us would meekly respond, "I am here," he would ask again more loudly.

"Where are you?" he would cry, prompting a student to match his volume. "Assert your presence in the space, in the room, and in this moment!"

"I am here!" they would finally shout back.

While the instructor was not speaking directly to me most of the time, I found myself becoming more emboldened to take up space within the room. At first, I played softly, focusing on holding the tall drum correctly and matching the beat exactly.

However, as our teacher repeatedly asked where we were, I closed my eyes and allowed myself to concentrate not only on what I was doing, but where I was and what it meant to be there.

Where am I? I asked myself.

I am here, in Ghana, I replied.

Are you? Are you sure? I challenged myself.

I let my drum speak for me as I played as hard as I could.

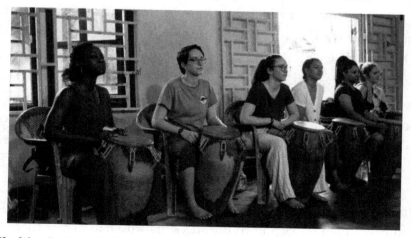

Khalila (left) and the other Ghana trip participants play the drums
Photo credit: LaToya Brackett, PhD

213

In that moment, I found myself deeply grounded by the feeling of my hands striking the drums and the ensuing vibration running through my fingers and down my arms. My heartbeat began to quicken and my eyes started to water as I reached a deeper understanding of what he was asking of us: *Make your presence known. Not just here, but everywhere.*

I thought back to my dance classes in which I had constantly felt I worried about how I would be perceived. In this moment, I was being given an opportunity to decide whether I would continue that old behavior or start choosing to show up entirely, facing my fear of standing out—even if there were potential consequences. This didn't just mean expressing myself here in the dance class; it meant being more authentic in my conversations, in my work as a clinician, and in the way I carried myself physically, both in Ghana and in the United States.

I will not hide anymore, I promised myself.

My new commitment would be tested in the dance portion of the class. Despite being surrounded by people who might have judged me, I decided I would exist in the here and now, paying attention not only to the dance being taught, but to how it made me feel. I would let those emotions shine through my movement, and not hide my artistic expression.

After the instructor had shown us the moves, he signaled to the drummers. As they began playing, I gave myself permission to follow the rhythm and flow with the music. I did not want to let this occasion go by without fully experiencing it or expressing myself. The drums helped make this possible: I could not only hear them; I could *feel* them. The drummers played with such power that my skin vibrated. I also noticed a reverberation in my heart. This music seemed to awaken every part of me, and I danced to celebrate that aliveness.

As I continued to move, I realized the sound and sensation of the drums were giving me a sense of peace and connection to the instruments themselves and to my ancestors who had played them for generations. I used this sense of groundedness to drive my movement. I stomped my feet and let my hips sway, dancing without fear that I would be seen as inappropriate or too sexy.

"African dance is intended to be expressed with the entire body!" our teacher told us when the song ended. "The legs, the feet, the arms, the hands, the chest, the hips—all of it! Fast or slow, staccato or legato: it's all correct when performed with intention."

After the class, based on the acknowledgement I received from my peers, I realized that my previous dance training had prepared me to perform the movements well. To my surprise, however, I did not put as much weight on my companions' affirmations as I would have before. I had simply wanted to enjoy learning and dancing. This was a level of freedom I hadn't experienced in a very long time.

As I looked around at the instructors who all resembled me, I also realized that being in Ghana felt different than spending time in predominantly Black and Brown spaces in the United States. Here, I knew that outside the four walls of any building, I was still in the majority. There was no entitled, unappointed "other" waiting to judge me for any mistake or for my mere existence.

As this awareness washed over me, I felt a warming sense of calm and relief. I realized that I could travel where I liked without feeling like all eyes were on me, and that I could peruse items in stores without the concern that someone would assume I was breaking the law. I knew I could dance in the way I felt inspired to, free of any worry about being pathologically sexualized because of the shape of my body or the way I moved.

My sense of this was confirmed when we went to a popular restaurant and karaoke bar that night for dinner. The crowd there was energetic and grooving to the upbeat music played by the DJ.

The vibe felt different to me than at most restaurants that cater to white customers in the United States. Rather than just sitting at their tables and listening to the music, the patrons swayed as they ate, and stood and danced by their seats when they felt moved. If they were really feeling it, they would head to the dance floor. People sang along to songs they knew when they heard them played by the DJ or performed on the karaoke stage.

While this had often been my experience in Black and Brown communities in the United States, I'd never been abroad in a country where this was the norm. I loved watching all the women here – who had curves like mine or were curvier – twist and sway on the dance floor. Seeing them, I knew that when I was inspired to get up and dance, I would be comfortable. I felt that there wouldn't be judgment about the fact that I had chosen to dance, the way I moved, or how my body was built.

***

Not all our experiences in Ghana were as pleasant as the dance class or that night out. The day that Professor Brackett prepared the trip leaders for the students' upcoming visit to Elmina Castle, the last place thousands of enslaved African people had seen before they were forcibly taken from their homeland, was difficult.

To make sure we would be ready to mentor the students during their visit, Professor Brackett invited us to go to the castle the day before. She thought it was important that we have the space and time to react without the students' eyes on us.

I will never forget descending into one of the dark, dank stone dungeons: I was overcome with emotion, taken aback by the drastic shift to stale air. I felt devastated as I tried to consider what it must have been like for my ancestors to be trapped there for months at a time. Picturing this devastating scene in the place it had occurred, I didn't just cry. I sobbed uncontrollably.

The somber feeling that developed during the tour didn't leave me until we explored the roof of the castle. We stood outside, breathing the fresh air as we looked over the town of Elmina. All of a sudden, I heard the sound of drums being played nearby. While I didn't think much could lift my spirits, the rhythmic beat forced me to concentrate on the music, rather than on the pain of this experience. I felt safe and reassured, just as I had in the dance class.

The following day, Professor Brackett divided the students into three racial affinity groups: Black, non-Black students of color, and white. Based on her previous scholarship and visits to Ghana, Professor Brackett had noted that different demographics have varied emotional reactions and questions while visiting the slave castles. The racial affinity groups were intended to provide the most conducive atmosphere for people to safely explore their emotions, fears, motivations, and biases in a way that could increase their self-awareness.

Touring the castle with the Black affinity group was a heavy experience, even though I had already been there the night before. Upon leaving, we boarded the bus and went to pick up our counterparts, who were visiting another castle nearby. As we traveled along, the mood began to lighten.

I overheard students lost in discussion about what they'd just seen and learned, as well as other, more everyday topics. Meanwhile, Professor Brackett and I talked about the phenomenon of Black resilience.

"It's incredible how our ancestors, and even the students now, can tap into joy while working through the depth of the moment," I said.

"I believe this is a major reason our people survived the atrocities we have faced for hundreds of years," Dr. Brackett responded.

As the bus made its way along the seaside road, I thought back to dance class the first day, our night out dancing and singing, and the way I'd felt when I'd heard the drums from the top of the castle.

"I think some music is in order," I said to Professor Brackett.

"That's a great idea," she replied, smiling.

"Abeiku!" I called our bus driver's name. By this point, he had become like another member of the group. "Do you happen to have a microphone? And can you play some Mary J. Blige, please?"

He chuckled softly, likely wondering what I was up to, as he handed me the microphone and turned on the music.

As I began to karaoke loudly and with vigor, the students roared with laughter and joined in. Standing there, I was expressing myself in a way that was truly authentic, lively and spontaneous, devoid of the seemingly incessant internal turmoil that had plagued me for years. The bliss that I felt in that moment was nothing less than magical.

When I offered the microphone to the students, they obliged. For the rest of that ride, they chose the songs. We heard music by City Girls and other modern Black artists I did not recognize.

Professor Brackett and I smiled and laughed as the students became more relaxed and engaged in the moment. As I watched them sing and dance, I felt warmth spread throughout my body. The power of being surrounded by people who can witness your self-expression without judgment, I recognized, is a healing experience that provides you with a sense of unity. This had been missing from my own artistic experiences, and now here I was providing a safe space for young Black people.

"After being here in Ghana, it may be a difficult transition back to life in the United States," Professor Brackett said, as the joyful scene continued to unfold. "Moments like these don't always feel accessible when you're in the minority and worried about how people could judge you."

"I definitely see what you mean," I responded. "We always talk about the frustration that comes with suppressing seemingly random urges to express ourselves due to fears of discrimination. Having to question ourselves and modify our behavior in public when we get back, just to make other people comfortable, is going to feel unbearable."

As I watched each student, I realized I never could have predicted how intense the impact of this trip would be. I felt more comfortable in my body and in my day-to-day existence than I had in a long time. Here, I was experiencing what it meant to act like myself without concern. And, while I could appreciate that my behavior had developed as a defense to keep me safe, I realized continuing with those habits would mean I was not really living, but just getting by. I was ready for something different.

***

I wish I could say that I had committed to live differently while in Ghana and—*poof*—it had worked. When I got home, however, I quickly saw that the next step of sharing myself more openly would be a challenge. I was now back in a country where Black self-expression was *not* completely accepted, and where I was *not* the majority outside any four walls.

Overwhelmed by the magnitude of my emotions, I did not leave my house for a few days. The idea of being surrounded by whiteness, and once again being pressured to censor what I said or did, was devastating. While I loved my home in the Pacific Northwest, I didn't want to lose how it felt to experience myself as I had in Ghana.

I knew the first real test of my conviction would be when my colleagues asked about the trip. The truth was that I didn't want to talk about it. I was still processing, and felt that most people would not be able to emotionally handle or contextually grasp the depth and complexity of my response. I was also aware that my answer could prompt feelings of guilt, shame, and possibly resentment from many white listeners, while also triggering my past trauma.

Luckily, when I finally went out to buy groceries, the first person I ran into was my boss, Dr. Kelly Brown, the first Black female director of Counseling, Health, & Wellness Services at the University of Puget Sound.

I called to her as I hurried across the parking lot.

"Hello, Khalila!" she exclaimed. "You must have just gotten back! It must be a really difficult transition for you."

I paused, speechless. She had recognized the gravity of what I had been through and what I was currently experiencing. I didn't have to explain, and I was grateful for it. Her immediate, unprompted empathy almost brought me to tears.

"It *is* difficult," I said, after a few moments. "I don't know if I'm ready to tell people about the trip, and I don't know if they are prepared to hear what I have to say. While I was in Ghana, I realized how much I've been holding myself back, and that I don't want to do that anymore."

"What if we talked it through together?" she offered.

"That would be great," I said. "Would you be open to giving me feedback on my prepared statement before I present it at the staff meeting?"

While the idea of speaking to a group about my time abroad made me very nervous, it was what I wanted, and it needed to be done. Dr. Brown agreed to my request, and we hugged before going our separate ways.

***

A few days later, I met with Dr. Brown and 14 other members of our predominantly white staff in a spacious, light-filled room. The tables were arranged in a square, with all of us facing the center so we could see each other.

Dr. Brown had printed out an agenda, and right in the middle of it, I saw my name: "Khalila – Ghana trip update."

I sat in a haze of terror throughout the beginning of the meeting, sweating and barely listening to the other topics being discussed. As my time to speak grew closer, I considered whether I should back out and remain silent.

As I engaged in this internal debate, I was reminded of what it had been like to be in ballet class just before performing a new sequence, or how I had felt before speaking in my graduate school courses. I was a different person now. I could be here, fully, as my dance and drumming teachers had encouraged in Ghana.

When it was my time to present, I held fast to the notes that Dr. Brown and I had prepared. My hands shook slightly, yet I was committed to bringing my whole self to this moment. As everyone turned toward me, I knew I could hide the way I had in dance class so many times, or I could speak up, asserting my presence as I'd promised myself I would in Ghana. I thought back to the soothing vibration of the drums. Taking a deep breath, I began.

"What I am about to convey is going to be uncomfortable for me," I said. "I don't want to mince words, and I want to make sure I'm clear and genuine. If I don't communicate this, I'm stepping over my truth for everyone else's comfort. If I do that, I will not have validated my experience and my needs."

Then I spoke about my journey.

Recommended resources:

Gates, H. L., Jr. (2014, July 13). True or False: There Are No Black People in Argentina. Retrieved July 09, 2020, from https://www.theroot.com/true-or-false-there-are-no-black-people-in-argentina-1790876367

Glefe Youth Ghana. (2019). Youth Empowerment: Glefe Youth Ghana: Accra, Ghana. Retrieved July 14, 2020, from https://www.glefeyouthghana.org/

Gyasi, Y. (2017). Homegoing: A Novel. New York, NY: Vintage Books.

Luongo, M. T. (2014, September 12). Argentina Rediscovers Its African Roots. Retrieved July 09, 2020, from https://www.nytimes.com/2014/09/14/travel/argentina-rediscovers-its-african-roots.html

Monteiro, N. M., PhD, & Wall, D. J., PsyD. (September 2011). African Dance as Healing Modality Throughout the Diaspora: The Use of Ritual and Movement to Work Through Trauma. *The Journal of Pan African Studies*, 4(6). doi:10.1163/1872-9037_afco_asc_3171

Persaud, D. (2011). *Traditional Ghanaian Dance and Its Role in Transcending Western Notions of Community* (Thesis). Occidental College. Retrieved July 8, 2020, from https://scholar.oxy.edu/cgi/viewcontent.cgi?referer=https://duckduckgo.com/&httpsredir=1&article=1002&context=rrap_student

Sumpter, L. (2015, July 21). Sound Healing: How Drumming Improves Mental and Physical Health. Retrieved July 14, 2020, from https://reset.me/story/sound-healing-how-drumming-improves-mental-and-physical-health/

LIFE IS RHYTHM

Lisa Josefsson (Li Storm)

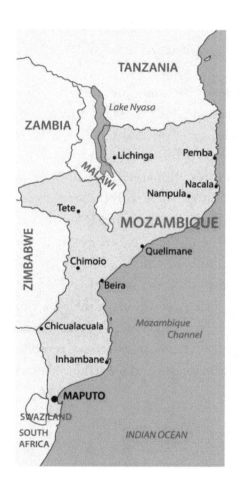

About the author: Lisa is an embodiment and sexuality coach who has explored, studied, and taught various dance styles for more than 15 years. Their research focuses on movement as a tool for healing, self-expression, and exploring our innate gender fluidity.

Lisa lived in Mozambique for three years, and has returned annually since 2015. Their time in the capital city of Maputo included extensive training in traditional dance with the Hodi Maputo Afro Swing performance company, as well as research on traditional emotional and sexual healing practices. Lisa now partners with Hodi to organize the annual Mozambique Afro Swing Exchange (MASX). Lisa's experience in Mozambique led them to create their own movement practice called Life Is Rhythm.

Based in Stockholm, Lisa's coaching program, "Dance into Your Lust," includes aspects of their learning in Africa, as well as dance and movement therapy, tantra, somatic experiencing, NARM, and motivational interviewing. To read more, visit www.masx.org and www.dancefromtheroot.com.

It's one o'clock in the morning, but it looks like midday. Light spills from the stores, restaurants, and giant video screens that line Times Square in New York City. As I make my way north on Seventh Avenue, I hear drums. I instinctively turn toward the rhythm and follow the sound.

The music gets louder and louder until, suddenly, it stops. I turn a corner to find three African American drummers packing up their belongings. They had not been playing drums, I realize, but rather buckets and pans of various sizes.

"Can you play again?" I ask politely. Noticing the hat they have out for tips, I add, "I'll pay! I know you will be good."

They smile back in agreement and pick up their drumsticks. As music fills the air once more, I feel it sink into my body. My shoulders, hips, and feet begin to move as if part of the ensemble. I make intense eye contact with each drummer as I follow his rhythm.

I feel the different beats inside of my body. As I dance, it seems as if ancient energies are flowing through me, and my body is their instrument. When the drumming is fierce, I channel a grounded masculinity, getting low and moving powerfully. My feet are steady on the ground, and I feel strong. When the music becomes playful, my sensual, feminine life force comes through, and I swirl my hips and torso to the rhythm. The percussionists and I are creating together, reacting to each other's inspiration. It is impossible to know who is leading and who is following. Each time one of us changes the dynamic, another part of me comes alive, eager to express itself.

When the musicians play the last break, I am sweaty and joyful. Looking around, I realize I've been dancing for almost an hour, and we've drawn a crowd.

"You've got some serious roots coming through," one of the drummers says to me. "Are you South African?" I understand why he would guess that a non-Black woman moving to the drums like this would be from South Africa, a country with a large white population.

"No," I respond. "I'm from Sweden."

"Sweden?" he asks, looking mystified. "But where did you learn to dance like that?"

"In Mozambique," I say, smiling.

***

In my home country, most people value hard work, planning, and efficiency. Two hundred years ago, we were farmers who lived off the land. Life was hard and required a forward-thinking mentality. In those times, during the long winters, everyone – especially the unprepared – risked starvation and death from exposure.

Over time, our society evolved. While life is now comfortable and stable for most people, the fear about the future persists in the form of a more existential struggle. There is an expectation that life needs to be perfect and must include a purposeful career, a nice house, a car, a spouse, children, and optimal health. This is an especially common attitude in the bigger cities like Stockholm and my hometown of Gothenburg.

As in many other Western countries, the desire for this way of life often leads to a fast-paced existence that does not always leave space for being present in the moment. Thus, there's less of an opportunity to cultivate qualities such as creativity, compassion, or vulnerability that may emerge when we slow down. Because of this, it's no surprise to me that burnout rates in many of these countries are rising.

I was an unknowing participant in the Swedish rat race for many years. Although I might not have had a typical day job, I packed my schedule with activities and to-dos. I embodied the hustle and ambition so esteemed by my peers as I diligently and naively worked toward my future goal: to make a difference in the world.

In Sweden, we are taught that our values, intelligence, and organizational skills are needed in developing countries, so many people decide to volunteer in Africa and other parts of the world. Unfortunately, most go there with the mindset that they're the only ones with something to offer, rather than the notion that they have a lot to learn.

***

At the age of 26, immersed in that bias, I arrived in Mozambique with a longing to contribute something meaningful. I'd come to the country to do research for my graduate thesis in economics. For three months, I would partner with a local NGO to interview children about the circumstances under which they fetched water and the amount of time it took them. I hoped the research would confirm my hypothesis that these chores affected their school results and attendance, and would raise awareness about the impact of the difficult water situation.

Though I wanted to do this work, I also had a deep desire to dance. I moved through each day with two parallel longings: an intellectual drive to make a difference, and a craving to feel the joy of moving with others to the sound of the drums. I would later discover that this longing was about more than dancing: it was about feeling something that was hard to experience in my own culture.

As I settled in, I found myself immersed in a way of life dramatically different than the one I'd known growing up. Everyone at the NGO, as well as the girls I shared a room with at the university campus, immediately treated me as if we were old friends. Rarely had I met people so openhearted, and seeing how much the Mozambicans valued community made me feel welcome.

Other parts of the culture were harder to adjust to. The pace of life was really slow. Even if someone was late, they would often prioritize taking their time getting ready or talking leisurely with a neighbor.

Around my new friends, I stood out. If I walked more quickly than my colleagues, they would say things like, "Relax! Why are you stressing yourself for no reason?"

When I rushed from place to place, people would also comment.

"Wow, you are walking so fast," they would say, laughing. "Where are you going that is so important?"

It was hard to take people's advice about loosening up, even though a part of me wanted to surrender to this different way of living. I was beginning to see that I had few other options, however. No matter what

227

I tried, I simply couldn't get as many things done as I had planned. It was frustrating. Before arriving, I'd imagined that my days would include visiting offices, doing my interviews, and having a fast lunch, so that I would still have time to study Mozambican traditional dance.

***

My enthusiasm for this art form began when I attended the Rock for Moc festival in Sweden at the age of 15. There, I had been lucky enough to see a show by the National Company of Song and Dance of Mozambique. The rhythms made me move in my seat, and the artists changed outfits for every dance! I loved all the colors of the fabrics, and especially the instrumental shakers made from leaves and seeds that the dancers tied to their legs. These adornments emphasized the rhythm of every step they took.

The performers were accompanied by several drummers, who struck their instruments with so much power that the air vibrated. There was also a musician playing the *timbila*, the traditional wooden xylophone that UNESCO has labeled a part of the Intangible Cultural Heritage of Humanity.[13] The timbila gave off an electrifying sound, making me wonder if there might be a synthesizer hidden nearby. I would later find out that this instrument was an important part of many traditional dances, such as Ngalanga and Semba.

My first opportunity to learn this art form came when my colleague and I visited the Department of Education to collect some documents I needed for my thesis work. Entering the building, we passed the broken elevator and headed up nine flights of stairs to the top floor.

In the office, the television was on, as is common in Mozambican workplaces. While most of the time, you see the news, local talk shows, or Brazilian soap operas, on this particular day, I saw a group of male dancers performing *Xigubo*. This warrior dance from the Changana tribe in the southern region of the country is similar to the South

---

[13] Chopi Timbila. (2008). Retrieved July 24, 2020, from https://ich.unesco.org/en/RL/chopi-timbila-00133

African *Indlamu* warrior dance done by the Zulus. Xigubo was traditionally a way for the men to build strength as they prepared for war. Today, it still helps people to build strength, stamina, and confidence, and is mainly performed as a celebration of peace.

The dancers on the show transitioned between slow, methodical movements accompanied by singing, and unbelievably fast, athletic dancing performed to drumming. They had on brown cow-leather skirts and carried wooden spears and shields. Long white tassels worn on their calves and upper arms accented their every jump, twist, and turn.

"I want to do that!" I told my colleague.

"I know a traditional performance group," he said. "They are incredible. I can introduce you."

The group's name was Wuchene (although the core artists have since founded a new dance company called Hodi Maputo Afro Swing), and they had regular practices at a primary school in the Polana Caniço B neighborhood.

The next day, I went to see them.

As I walked through the streets made of hard-packed, orange sand, I passed simple, unpainted concrete homes. Families relaxed in their front yards, smiling and laughing. Kids were everywhere, as were old women selling local produce. They sat on the ground, wearing a *capulana* (a colorful piece of African cloth) displaying their tomatoes, onions, and hot peppers. Some might have called this neighborhood poor. To me, it felt alive.

Approaching the school, I heard drumming. The sound was so loud that my chest vibrated as I entered the rehearsal space. It didn't take long for the dancers to notice my presence. Although they had no idea who I was, they greeted me with hugs and invited me to join their practice. I was delighted to participate.

Of course, they did not slow down to accommodate me. Swallowing my pride, I tried to follow the sets of ever-changing moves. As I danced, I felt rigid and confused next to my Mozambican counterparts, who had mastered the transitions and fluid, full-body extension to the lightning-fast music.

By the end of the practice, I felt both awkward and awestruck. I could sense my Swedish stiffness, and I thought I would never be able to dance with the beauty and power of these performers.

Afterwards, the group invited me to stay and watch them rehearse for an upcoming performance in Shanghai. The show began like most traditional rituals, with call-and-response singing. The artists' voices filled the space with male choral chanting. As strong, bare-chested men entered the room with determination, I could feel the masculine energy in the air. Even the skinniest, youngest ones displayed resolute confidence. As their final notes echoed into silence, the dancing began.

The movements – the same I'd seen on TV just one day earlier – were mesmerizing. The men jumped, kicked, and spun their way through the space, moving with the athletic prowess of the countless warriors who had lived before them. By the time the drummers played the final break in the music, I had goosebumps.

Why aren't these artists out touring the world? I wondered. I was sitting in a dusty school in the suburbs, feeling like I was watching a Broadway performance.

As weeks went by, I was amazed to learn that the Hodi artists could do around 25 traditional dances from different tribes around the country. My new friends explained to me that each of the pieces shared a story from the elders, expressed different emotions, and recounted important moments in history. In this way, the vast wisdom of Mozambican culture was passed on to each generation.

In addition to Xigubo, there was *Ngalanga*, which expresses pure joy and flirtatious human connection; *Nganda*, a depiction of the authority of the Portuguese colonizers; the harvest dance *Tema Tema*, exemplifying the movements of workers in the fields, and many others.

They also did Mozambique's most famous dance, *Marrabenta*, which was popularized in the 1940s when it had united Mozambicans and Portuguese youngsters in the city nightclubs of Maputo. Marrabenta has many sensual and playful moves, and is just as popular today as it was back then. In fact, many new artists have produced more modern versions of the music.

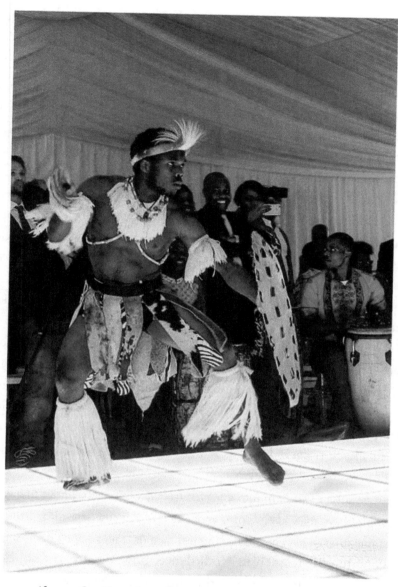

Alexandre Soquisso from Hodi Maputo Afro Swing
dances Xigubo at a wedding in Maputo
Photo credit: Alex Manguele

Each time Hodi performed, I was overwhelmed by their energy and presence. To my surprise, I saw this not only when they danced, but also in our other interactions. Their behavior was a stark contrast to my own, as it was not easy for me to express myself and my emotions openly at that time.

Growing up, I'd been taught not to stand out or be "too much." In Sweden, we even have an old, traditional code of conduct called *Jantelagen* (the Law of Jante), which stresses adherence to the collective over individuality. This mindset might be good when you want to follow societal norms and create a stable life, but it hinders self-expression and self-actualization.

Though I didn't know it at the time, my dependence on my intellect and underdeveloped emotional intelligence blocked my ability to move in an authentic way. Because I could not let go of control, I could not surrender to the true meaning of each dance and honor the different parts of myself the way the other artists could. Thus, my performances lacked the aliveness and expression of my Mozambican counterparts.

Marrabenta was particularly challenging for me, since I'd never valued sensuality. In fact, I'd grown up with the idea that a woman dancing in a sensual way was objectifying herself to get attention from men. When I would do the moves to this rhythm, my Mozambican girlfriends would constantly tell me I wasn't being feminine enough. Their feedback triggered me, as it went against the feminist mindset I had developed as a teenager.

Just because I was born into a female body doesn't mean I have to buy into traditional gender roles like wearing makeup and dancing sensually, I thought. That's something women only do to impress men as a result of chauvinism.

Watching the women in Hodi dance, however, I had to question my beliefs. For example, when the drummers played Zorre - which Hodi's female dancers said was the most empowering women's dance from the region - the ladies expressed so much joy and pride in shaking their hips that I longed to feel the way they did.

When I asked the men why the women danced Zorre, they said, "It's to show off their beauty and seduce us."

When I mentioned this to the women, they laughed and said, "That is what they think, but we do it because it makes us feel so good!"

***

One night, I joined my friends at a dance club in downtown Maputo, where a DJ was playing South African house music that went straight into your core, awakening your hips. I found my flow and danced with a guy who was both very skilled and incredibly present. We mirrored each other's movements and played off one another. At times it seemed like we were one: I felt powerful in what I can now say was a masculine way.

The atmosphere on the floor continued to build, and a jam circle formed. The first person to enter was the man I had just danced with. A woman in a long, red dress soon joined him. She was tall and moved gracefully as she approached the man with an aura of confidence. I could feel that she knew her full power, and I noticed I was jealous. The energy was different from when I had been partnered with the same person.

These two invited a polarity of the masculine and feminine that brought a palpable sensuality to the room. While people who are not familiar with the dance might have seen their connection and joint rhythmic hip movement as sexual, I knew from talking with the Hodi dancers that it was meant to be loving and playful. As I continued to watch, I realized I would have been too ashamed to allow myself to be seen in a similar way.

As the song came to an end, the woman turned around, bent down, and made a traditional twerking movement. With her last upward shake, she bumped the man's pelvis with her hips, and then walked off with pride. My friends' words echoed in my mind: "Dancing like that makes us feel good!"

At that moment, I felt inspired. Perhaps it *was* worth exploring a similar energy within myself. I now saw how it could be valuable to embrace the feminine, as the ladies in Hodi had encouraged me to. After all, this woman had owned the room in a way I had not known was possible, and I could feel the respect and appreciation the crowd was exuding for her. Here, I realized, a woman expressing herself

233

sensually while dancing could be part of feminism, since it made her feel empowered.

That night, and many other moments, would help me see that my Mozambican friends were more in touch with the full range of humanity that lives within us all. To embrace one's innate sensual energy was natural, and women and men in this country seemed able to enjoy it more freely. Through traditional dances, this way of connecting was celebrated and passed down from generation to generation.

Because the Mozambican relationship to sensuality stood in such stark contrast to what I'd known in my own life, I now understood the extent to which many people in northern European white cultures have been shamed about their innate sexual drive. I could see that this has become a transgenerational trauma. Furthermore, I was starting to believe that my resentment of femininity had cut me off from part of my identity and limited my ability to feel pleasure. Even when I longed to be in contact with this part of myself, I did not feel free to express it.

***

As I observed this all further, it became clear to me that people's ability to embrace all parts of themselves through rhythm and to derive satisfaction from life in general were truly linked.

This became clear to me when I joined my friends in singing and dancing at a colleague's father's funeral. They were simultaneously sharing their sadness with the community and celebrating someone's life. Over and over again, I saw how music and movement helped Mozambicans move through both their highs and lows without becoming attached to either. It was a way of life that permeated all parts of their experience.

This also helped me better understand certain interactions I'd had with Hodi's dancers that had previously perplexed me. Once, after practice, I had walked home with a colleague who told me that he was hungry because he hadn't been able to afford to eat that day. At the time, I hadn't been able to understand how he'd managed to dance joyfully and energetically for hours. Now, I could see that he'd just embraced the circumstances and continued his day as planned, with or without food.

Another time, after seeing a dancer perform powerfully, I heard that his brother had passed away.

"Staying at home and being sad with my family would have made me feel worse," he would tell me later. "I decided I might as well go to practice, where my friends would be there to support me." It was evident to me now that rhythm and dance in this context could be therapeutic.

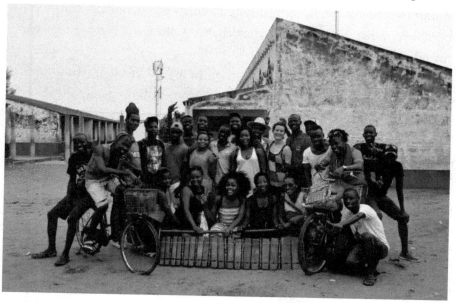

The author with the members of Hodi in the neighborhood of Polana Caniço in Maputo Photo credit: Hanna Turesson Bernhed

As these insights into wellbeing, rhythm, and life became clearer, I became more decisive about facing my own struggles. I found solace in knowing that my goal was bigger than just learning to dance.

Therefore, even though I still felt self-conscious about not moving as smoothly as my Mozambican counterparts, I continued to practice. As the weeks passed, I stopped trying to figure out each step in my head. To dance with more fluidity, authenticity, and self-expression, I had to let the drums move me instead of trying to be in control.

Now I was exploring many new parts of myself that I'd unconsciously repressed. I learned that I could be humble and soft, rather than just strong and powerful, and I realized how good it felt to move my body in new ways. It was liberating and invigorating to discover how to make each dance my own.

The movement, the rhythm, and the Hodi community became impossible to leave behind. My experience in Maputo became so profound that my three-month stay evolved into years of traveling between Mozambique and Sweden. As these visits became an ever-greater part of my life, my conditioned beliefs and behaviors slowly grew more apparent, and my idea that there is always a right and wrong started to dissipate.

The aspects of local culture that had bothered me in Maputo started to make sense. Suddenly, I could enjoy walking really slowly and taking time to speak to friends I might encounter on my way, even when I was late for something else. I could also appreciate the gift of alone time when I had to wait for someone, understanding that they probably had a good reason for not having arrived yet. Each culture, I now understood, has both wonderful and challenging aspects. Seeing the stress and lack of presence in many people on the streets of Stockholm was a reminder that no way of being is inherently better than any other.

I could laugh now when I thought about how some Swedish people had been annoyed with my change of behavior the last time I had been home. It was worth it. Not only did I feel more relaxed, but I found that ecstatic dancing moments were coming into my life in new ways.

***

One of my most memorable nights in Mozambique came about three years after my first visit. That evening, I went out by myself to Nucleo de Arte, my favorite club for dancing.

Every Sunday, people from across the city head to this venue to enjoy music played by various live African bands. As you walk through the building, you discover an almost hidden art gallery full of traditional and modern African paintings and sculptures. Among the colorful landscapes and drawings of proud African women, you can also find eye-catching statues. These works were created by the famous artist, Mabunda, out of old weapons from Mozambique's civil war.

Outside, a bounty of colorful lights hangs over a small dance floor, keeping the discothèque spirit alive. The space is always packed with Mozambicans and foreigners, old and young. Everyone has a place somehow, and as soon as you encounter the crowd, you feel like you are part of a community. People smile and welcome you. And the rhythm! The beats are so irresistible that your body automatically starts to move.

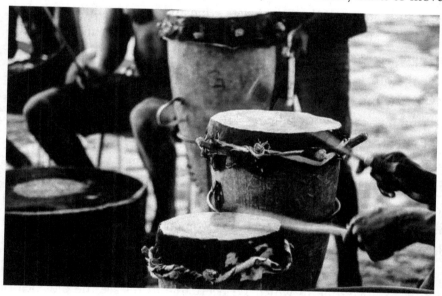

Hodi Musicians playing todje drums
Photo credit: Sanna Greneby

On that particular night, I heard the unique sound of a timbila ringing out as a professional drummer flawlessly stacked Ngalanga rhythms on top of the music. A hallmark of this traditional dance from the Chope tribe is the shaking, and the two people dancing (most commonly, a woman and a man) will face each other and grow increasingly ecstatic as they shake their hips and upper bodies to the rhythm.

A jam circle had formed, and new pairs were entering as they felt called. They showed their spirit and best steps, and the crowd cheered as magical moments of movement and music came together. Everyone on the dance floor was engaged. The band members were fully with us, and the lead drummer followed the dancers' body language as if it had all been choreographed. I felt a growing desire to step into the circle.

And then, suddenly, I was there.

I was not thinking; my body just knew what to do. I looked into the eyes of my dance partner, a tall, handsome man with dreadlocks whom I had encountered several times. We communicated through our movements and facial expressions, playing off each other, and I felt more and more as if the crowd were gone and we were alone.

The man had an intense presence, but I was not intimidated. I was energized, and grounded in the music. I shook that Ngalanga dance like never before, as if I were releasing generations of tension from my body. My chest and butt popped back and forth at an incredible speed, making my whole body vibrate. The rhythm was guiding me, and my movements, in turn, were inspiring the musicians.

As our dance approached its end, the drummer was ready for the final Ngalanga rhythm break, and so was I. Not only did I use the traditional twerking movement, but I grabbed my partner and humped him from behind as I'd seen other women do many times before. I didn't just do it once; I almost chased him off the dance floor.

When the Ngalanga rhythm finished, I felt like I had been ripped out of a trance—one in which I'd been able to release the old idea of who I could be and connect to an undiscovered part of myself. A tickling sensation ran through my body.

As the shock of the moment wore off, I realized the crowd was cheering and whistling wildly. I was excited, blushing, and shaking from having unleashed so much of myself. I felt vulnerable... but I was also in a state of absolute bliss from having allowed the power within me to come alive. I wanted more.

One man came up to me and said, "Wow, you really feel it. It is great to see a woman like you honoring our culture in this way."

The Hodi artists have told me the same thing many times since.

Whenever I doubt my abilities, they say I shouldn't give up, and that I honor their heritage by understanding their connections to each other and to life.

While Mozambican traditional dances were discriminated against and even forbidden at times during colonialism, they have never been appropriated. Because of this, people in Mozambique generally don't fear the idea of foreigners "stealing" their art forms. As long as a performer does the dance well and gives proper credit to its originators, most Mozambicans feel that this helps spread a positive image of their country. This is why I always share my respect for the Mozambicans' cultural heritage, and talk about my teachers as the experts. I see myself as a "cultural bridge" as I discuss what I have learned to embody. If there were no bridges, everyone would stay on their separate islands.

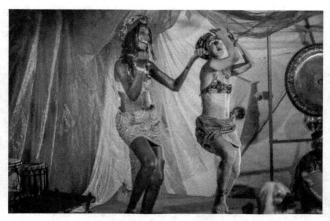

Lisa and their dear friend, Hallazy Manhice, dancing Zorre at the Borderland festival in Denmark
Photo credit: Yann Houlberg Andersen

***

I'd gone to Maputo hoping that I would "change the world." This had meant that, unconsciously, I regarded the values from my Swedish upbringing so highly that I believed them to be superior to anyone else's. It had hurt to realize this, as I'd had to come to terms with a certain arrogance on my part. In the end, it was my own world that shifted, and

239

my thesis was never even published.

Through my experiences in Mozambique, I was given a whole new family. Whenever I leave the country, my friends say, *"Você já é nossa!"* ("You are already ours!") I feel that, too, and I know that one part of my heart will always be with them.

My time there gave me a different way of being and living, too. Now, as I work with somatic movement and study trauma healing, I am fascinated by how closely modern research and methods align with my lived experience in Mozambique, and I see more and more evidence that trying to control life will not result in a healthy rhythm.

It frightens me to think about where I would be today if I hadn't gone on that first trip to Maputo. I would likely have burned out, as so many of my friends and colleagues have. Instead, I began a therapeutic, healing journey that has continued to this day. Whether I am walking through the streets of Stockholm, or dancing to bucket drummers in New York City, I embrace my new philosophy: life is rhythm.

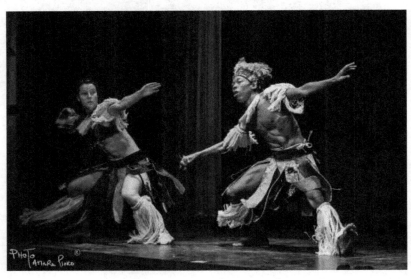

Lisa and Paulo Inácio dance Xigubo in 2014 at
Herrang Dance Camp in Herrang, Sweden
Photo credit: Tamara Pinco

Acknowledgments: *I want to thank all the dancers and musicians from*

Hodi Maputo Afro Swing, who are always by my side: Elias Manhiça, Eugénio Macuvel, Judite Novela, Sonia Vembane, Luisa Nhaca, Victoria Matangala, Roda Cossa, Erzenia Tamele, Delfina Godo, Macario Natu, Vasco Sitoe, Paulo Inácio, Alexandre Soquisso, Vasco Uate, Nilegio Cossa, Augusto Manhica, Fernando Sitoe, Manuel Manhica, Jossefa Macuacua, Robath Kunuma, Inácio Ubisse, and Manuel Zita. Thank you, too, to our padrinho, (godfather), Juma, who lovingly supports our dance company, as well as to my dear sister, Halaze Manhice, who catches me when I fall. I want to thank my madrinha (godmother), Angela Andrew, for pushing me to admit my mistakes and encouraging me to constantly strive to be a better version of myself. Thank you to my mentor, Mickey Davidsson Aduke, for always seeing the heart in my work and believing in me through my ups and downs. Last but not least, without the love and support from my family, Hans, Iréne, and Gustaf, this journey would not have even started.

Recommended resources:

Baskerville, N. (2014). *Twerk It: Deconstructing Racial and Gendered Implications of Black Women's Bodies Through Representations of Twerking* (Unpublished master's thesis). Swarthmore College. Retrieved July 23, 2020, from
https://scholarship.tricolib.brynmawr.edu/bitstream/handle/10066/14354/Baskerville_thesis_2014.pdf?sequence=1&isAllowed=y

Hodi Maputo Afro Swing • Mozambique Afro Swing Exchange • 5th Anniversary • Lindy Hop AFRICA. (2019, January 12). Retrieved July 07, 2020, from https://masx.org/what-is-afro-swing/hodi-maputo-afro-swing/

Mahlasela, V. (Director). (2018, July 5). *Say Africa (Live)* [Video file]. Retrieved July 7, 2020, from https://www.youtube.com/watch?v=LlOmPo48vCI

Pauladas, M. (Producer). (2018, February 9). *Gemeos Manhica*

Sizodivana by MZV Filmes FullHD VIDEO OFFICIAL [Video file]. Retrieved July 7, 2020, from https://www.youtube.com/watch?v=RozCgo-GbsY

Seandulac (Poster). (2007, June 18). *Music and Life - Alan Watts* [Video file]. Retrieved July 7, 2020, from https://www.youtube.com/watch?v=ERbvKrH-GC4

Theleaders-Online. (2019, July 11). Rwandan Prescription for Depression: Sun, Drum, Dance, Community. Retrieved July 23, 2020, from https://theleaders-online.com/rwandan-prescription-for-depression-sun-drum-dance-community/

INTER-INDEPENDENCE

Zsuzsi Kapas

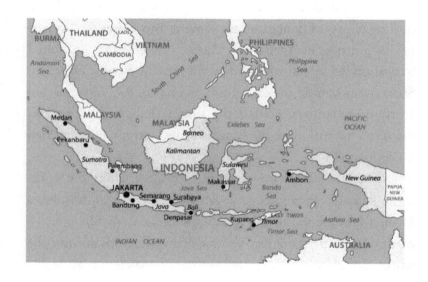

About the author: Zsuzsi is a Hungarian who was born in the former Czechoslovakia. Her family immigrated to the United States in 2000 to leave behind a life of ethnic oppression. In the following pages, Zsuzsi shares a story from her three-year journey around the world, during which she studied the healing effects of dance and movement improvisation. As part of this journey, in April 2017, Zsuzsi traveled to Java to join a workshop led by improvisational movement mentor Suprapto Suryodarmo, more widely known as Prapto. As Prapto passed away on December 29, 2019, this story is dedicated to him and the immense influence his Amerta Movement practice has had on so many lives.

Zsuzsi is based in Los Angeles, CA, USA, where she works as a somatic movement, yoga therapy, and mindfulness facilitator at mental health rehabilitation centers. She is also a certified aquatic therapist who has led workshops around the world. Zsuzsi holds a BS in behavioral neuroscience, an MBA, and an advanced certificate in somatic psychotherapy. For more information visit: www.embodiedartoflife.com.

I proudly scanned the crisp, white page where my good grades were noted in the blue swirls of my teacher's cursive handwriting. Sitting in the front row of the classroom, I attentively reviewed every word, feeling satisfied with my accomplishments. Alongside me, my fellow second graders were looking over their own report cards.

The teacher had used the Slovakian version of my name: Zuzana Kapasova. I had learned to accept this modification of my real name, Zsuzsi Kapas, since the change had been made for legal documentation purposes. This adjustment of Hungarians' names was standard practice in postwar Czechoslovakia. At a time when Slovaks discriminated against Hungarians, we forced ourselves to go along with these modifications. Although changing our names made us cringe, we knew it ultimately protected us from further abuse or exploitation.

Everything I saw on my report card met my expectations, except for one thing: my teacher had entered my nationality as Slovak. Unlike my name, the choice of how I listed my nationality was still up to my family. My parents always made sure we wrote that we were Hungarian, since pride in our heritage was one of the only things no one could take away. Our identity, culture, and commitment to high moral standing were things no one could touch.

I raised my hand.

"Yes, Zuzana?" my teacher said.

"Excuse me," I responded in the proper manner, standing up as I'd been taught to do whenever a teacher called on me. "There is incorrect information on my report card. It says my nationality is Slovak, not Hungarian. I need this corrected before I take it home."

"Let it be, Zuzana," my teacher told me. "It is better for your future this way."

Anger coursed through me. Being misrepresented like this felt like losing one of the last things I could control.

I imagine myself there now: a blonde seven-year-old with a short, boyish haircut doing her best to stand up for herself. I was likely wearing corduroy pants the color of freshly baked bread and a white blouse with burgundy polka dots. I had worn this hand-me-down outfit often over the years, my mom letting down the hem at the bottom of the pants each time I had a growth spurt. I knew exactly how many times she'd done that. I could count the creases that no amount of ironing seemed to smooth out. We had to reuse everything we could in order to save money. It was very common for Hungarians to live in poverty at that time, as much of our property had been stolen and redistributed to Slovaks.

Ultimately, my report card stayed the same. Something else did change, however. Now that I had made my ethnicity clear, my peers began the harassment common against Hungarians at the time. Each day, my classmates would push me, trip me, or steal my school supplies. Several made it their mission to destroy my school projects before I could turn them in. My teacher did not help me, since I had not heeded her advice to hide my nationality.

This experience marked a notable shift in my life. From then on, I would hide the parts of my identity I loved most. Otherwise, I thought, they would be ruined, ridiculed, or taken away from me.

Over the next few years, I gathered more evidence that this was true. I watched my family and friends experience hurt, betrayal, and suffering in numerous ways simply because they were Hungarian. Reveal who you are and what you love most, it seemed, and there would always be a negative result. This fear and trauma manifested in a habit of hiding who I was, as well as in chronic pain throughout my body.

***

At the age of 16, when I moved to the United States, I continued to conceal much of my life from others. After discovering a passion for dance, I did not commit myself to a career in this field, knowing my family would not approve. Instead, I studied neuroscience and organizational development, and later took a job in the corporate world.

I kept my love for the expressive arts hidden, not knowing that one day, it would be movement improvisation that would hold the key to my healing. Still, I was starting to long to be seen and known for who I was—even if this felt uncomfortable.

Over the next several years, I found just one person I could open up to: a woman named Jordyn, who became my best friend. Jordyn was also a dancer, so I felt comfortable embracing my identity as an artist when we were together. She seemed to have endless energy, and delighted in creative expression of all kinds. I felt inspired by how lovingly she treated everyone, from friends to perfect strangers. We enjoyed talking about poetry and costume-making, and spent hours chatting by the pool.

I could write extensively about my growing friendship with Jordyn, my exploration of different types of dance, and more. For now, however, I will simply say that two profound events led me to think about creating a life that was very different than the one I had built.

The first was that the chronic pain I'd developed as a child intensified to the point that it was unbearable. I was experiencing migraines and a loss of sensation in my fingers and toes. Often, a sharp, lightning-bolt shot of pain would move through my body, causing uncontrollable spasms and convulsions.

My 12-hour days at the office made it all worse. Because I was holding still as I worked, I would go home every day in pain, having lost significant range of motion and mobility. To manage this, I created a morning and evening practice in which I would do yoga, meditate, and allow my body to unwind through improvised movement. Inspired, I enrolled in a somatic movement training offered through a yoga center, and began to devote more of my time to these types of practices.

I did not, however, find the courage to devote myself fully to dance until April 1, 2013, the day of the second event. Up until this time, I was still in an internal battle with myself. I'd invested so much money and time in my schooling. I had a prestigious career. Was I really going to start all over?

Sometimes it takes a terrible experience to jolt us out of indecision. That morning, I learned Jordyn had taken her own life. It was a shock to me and everyone who knew her. We would find out later about the pain and childhood trauma that had driven her to this act.

Jordyn had lived a life dedicated to the things she loved, and with her passing, I knew it was time for me to do the same. I could no longer treat dance as a hobby, both because of my passion and because I needed to heal my chronic pain.

Ready for change in my life and career, I left the United States and began traveling through Europe and Asia. In each location, I took workshops and apprenticed with teachers who would help me explore self-expression through relational movement practices. I saw this as critical to my preparation for my new vocation.

I had dozens of fantastic and transformative experiences during this period, but none would impact me as much as my time in Indonesia. The next part of this story begins with my arrival in the city of Surakarta (colloquially called Solo) in Central Java.

***

As my plane descended, I admired the deep blue ocean. I had been daydreaming about coming to Solo since a woman I'd met in Thailand had told me about her studies in Java. There, she had worked with renowned improvisational movement mentor Suprapto Suryodarmo, more widely known as Prapto.

I later learned that, since 1970, Prapto had developed his unique approach called Joged Amerta based on his study of free movement, Vipassana, and Javanese Sumarah meditation techniques. His workshops were often held at historical and cultural sites in Indonesia and throughout the world.

What I'd heard about Amerta Movement fascinated me. This form of dance recognizes both the importance of the individual and the universal spirit that moves through every living thing. Most of Prapto's workshops were held not in recital halls, but in public spaces and at heritage sites to allow for an energy exchange ritual between a practitioner and the outside world. For example, a person might move with vigor and joy, offering energy to onlookers. In return, she would receive her audience's emotional reaction. This would then inform what came next. Amerta Movement thus encouraged an organic, in-the-moment creation.

I rented a room at a homestay 30 minutes from the Wisma Seni Public Arts Center of Solo, where Prapto would guide his workshop for the next few days. The homestay room was dark and basic. The bed was hard, and the bathroom had a well with cold water for bucket showers. Confronted by the harsh intensity of city life, I found I was balancing deep concern for my physical health with immense gratitude for the opportunity to study with Prapto. With my chronic pain and overactive immune system, I worried my body wouldn't be able to withstand the noise, water, and air pollution. I felt deeply that I was meant to be here, however, so I set an intention to care for myself as best I could throughout the experience.

The next morning, I rented a scooter and rode through chaotic traffic to the entrance of the arts center. Prapto was in a small restaurant there, ordering breakfast and smoking a *kretek* clove cigarette. He was in his 70s, had long, grey hair, and was wearing a black, loose-fitting Javanese outfit.

I walked over and introduced myself. Prapto invited me to join him, so I sat down across the table. With no other students there to observe, I was unsure how to behave with him. I didn't know whether there was a special way to interact with teachers in Java, and I did not want to accidentally overstep. To be safe, I ordered a cup of tea and waited silently for Prapto to address me first.

Rather than talk, we simply sat silently and drank our tea together.

A short while later, another workshop participant arrived. She told me that it was her last day of practice, so I took her lead on how to interact with Prapto. The two were relaxed and friendly together. This would not, it seemed, be a hierarchical or rigid learning environment like many others I'd known.

After Prapto's breakfast, the three of us walked to Wisma Seni to begin our practice in its *pendopo*, a pillared, open pavilion that serves as a space for performances and social-cultural activities. It has a roof, but is open on four sides, which offers complete exposure to the surroundings. We would practice in this urban setting, breathing the pollution and hearing the traffic. Prapto seemed relaxed in the midst of it all. He sat on the dusty concrete, smoking one cigarette after another.

***

That first week, I learned that a typical workshop day had three distinct parts. Each morning, two participants from China, a woman from Finland, and I had a three-hour practice session. We would move without music, listening to and interacting with the sounds of the world. Afterward, over lunch, we would talk about what we had experienced while Prapto shared concepts from his Joged Amerta work. The day would end with a two-hour afternoon session during which we would try to incorporate the ideas from our discussion.

Prapto would sometimes join in. More often, however, he would sit off to the side, observe us, and speak, directing our awareness to areas of our body or our movement. Sometimes he would guide a specific person by saying their name and then following up with instructions. Other times, however, his suggestions seemed to be for everyone.

"Feet not be late," he once said as he watched us. I interpreted this as an invitation to integrate the pace of my feet with the impulse from my upper body.

"Voice—open the throat!" he called another day, and everyone in the pendopo began to create various sounds. Participants sang notes or chanted as they felt inspired to do so.

"Body having sound versus sound having body!" He then exclaimed. I used this as a cue to allow my movements to create the sound of my voice, rather than having my body react to the noises I made.

I played with incorporating all the prompts Prapto called out, but he never indicated whether I was following his directions correctly. I hoped he would eventually offer me personalized feedback, as I saw him do for others, but he never did.

Assuming this was part of the process, I stayed quiet. As the days went on, my mind grew increasingly busy. Did Prapto think I was doing everything correctly? Or was he forgetting to pay me the specific attention he was giving to the others? After three days, I was eager for clarification, and decided to talk with him.

After our morning practice, while the other dancers went to get their lunch, I approached Prapto. He was alternately taking bites of his lunch and drags on his cigarette.

"Pak Prapto!" I greeted him, using the respectful term *pak* (sir). "If you don't mind, I have some questions regarding my practice."

I couldn't tell if Prapto had heard me. He didn't make eye contact or respond. Unsure of what to do, I continued.

"I notice you sometimes call out instructions to the other dancers, but you haven't yet done that with me," I said. "Is this because I should be responding to your general suggestions, trying to work with the comments you're giving the others, or just going on with my own inquiry?"

Prapto said nothing.

"I would really like to make good use of my time here and improve in a focused way," I went on. "I'd love to hear your thoughts."

Without looking at me, Prapto responded, "You are depending too much on my validation."

I was surprised by his statement, and hurt by what I perceived as his judgment. I felt like I was being dismissed, just as I had in my second-grade classroom. He seemed to be disregarding what was important to me and treating me differently than my peers. I'd seen Prapto talk with others, and I knew he often gave them feedback.

The other dancers began returning to the pendopo with their food, and Prapto initiated our daily group discussion. When one woman from China asked a question, Prapto turned to her, smiling, and began a lively conversation.

My inner, wounded child struggled with a feeling of rejection. I wondered if Prapto was playing favorites, or if he simply approached everyone in a way that would serve them. I wanted to trust that, as my mentor, he was taking me on a journey that would help me grow. For this reason, I chose to see my upset as a sign that there was something for me to learn.

A few days later, at the morning session, Prapto asked us all to improvise a dance by interacting with various elements in our surroundings.

"Stop to find interesting," he instructed. "Space and time to say hello."

I closed my eyes to tune into my body and the surroundings. I felt the wind brush against my skin, offering direction to my movement. I relaxed so the currents could guide me into new shapes and in new directions. As the wind moved me to the edge of the floor, I noticed a swaying blade of grass. I took on its playful quality, enjoying the experience of being in sync with nature. Out of the corner of my eye, I spotted the edge of the wall. Immediately, I stiffened to greet it, bringing the sharpness of its structure into my shape. On I went, allowing myself to "say hello" to each object that caught my attention. As I matched the characteristics I observed in the world around me, I felt alive and safe. By taking on the qualities of the environment, I was trying to keep my own essential self from being seen and judged.

Then Prapto inserted an inquiry: "How to be with the 'I' that is connecting with the other organism?"

I paused, trying to understand what he meant. Was Prapto suggesting that I was not asserting my presence?

He continued, "You are not the grass, so why are you reducing yourself to act like grass?"

I continued to move in the pendopo, thinking back to how I'd been dancing so far. I was indeed becoming like the grass, the wall, or the other dancers around me, rather than co-creating with them from a place of my own solid being. This dynamic mirrored interactions in the rest of my life. In fact, this was exactly why I'd started my travels: I wanted to learn to fully express myself and to live with the authenticity that I craved.

Over lunch that day, Prapto introduced the concept of inter-independence. When a dancer practices inter-independence, he explained, she can interact with someone or something else without sacrificing her essential self. She does not renounce her internal sensations or external expression during this process, but instead maintains a sense of centeredness while organically discovering what unfolds as she comes in contact with this other entity.

I felt a wave of excitement move through me. It was as if a door had just opened. Amerta Movement was offering me a unique chance to cultivate the skills necessary for self-expression not only in my dancing, but also in my life. By practicing inter-independence, I would better learn to hear and honor my needs, inclinations, and desires in each moment.

Given how conditioned I was to conform, I decided on a first step. During the afternoon practice, I would give myself permission to focus solely on myself. That way, I could discover how I felt inspired to dance away from the influence of others. My existence would no longer be about avoiding conflict or confrontation. It would be about learning to express and stand up for myself.

After lunch, we entered the pendopo again.

How do you feel like dancing? I asked myself, directing my attention toward the floor. The inspiration for a slow, flowing practice came over me, and I surrendered to that desire, playing with different moves until I found a deep sense of satisfaction in my experience.

A few minutes later, the woman from China approached me. A professional dancer, she moved with refined precision. I felt my body grow alert to her presence and felt an impulse to show her she was welcome by altering my movement. Instead, I focused inward. Noticing I wasn't interacting with her, the woman danced away. Pangs of regret and isolation washed over me as I watched her go.

Over the next couple hours, the other dancers would sometimes come toward me. Rather than react, I continued to focus on my own movement and process the emotions that arose. I felt compassion for my younger self, who had never felt a true sense of acceptance and had been desperate to be seen, known, and validated.

I also noticed empathy for my current self: the older, wiser woman who was doing the painful work required to release old patterns, and using the dance floor as a way to stand up for her truth.

In the coming days, with each interaction, the pain dissolved into a dull ache, accompanied by a sense of groundedness. I felt thankful for my newfound boundaries, and no longer experienced an intense need to seek approval or change myself in the presence of others.

Each time I took a break, I would stand off to the side and watch Prapto dance, awed by his mastery of inter-independence. His movement was dynamic and unpredictable. He would move slowly, fast, alone, or in physical contact with others. Prapto entered and exited interactions with ease, and seemed to move through instinct. Although his face and body were expressive and constantly changing, he did not often smile. He seemed unburdened by any need to exhibit friendliness.

***

It was a chilly, rainy day when I finally felt centered enough to expand my awareness outward. After days of focusing solely on myself, I would now experiment with inter-independence.

As I entered the practice space, I felt the marble floor icy cold under my feet. The chill moved up through my body, settling into my bones. I knew moving quickly would warm me up, but I felt inspired to go slowly, wishing to start my practice by gently deepening my connection to myself.

I danced mindfully, intricately styling each movement and focusing on how it felt to be in my practice. Only after I was completely centered did I permit my focus to oscillate between my inner world and the world around me. I allowed myself to notice a pillar in the pendopo, raindrops, the wind, and the grass. More than ever before, I could acknowledge their presence without disturbing my internal equanimity.

After about an hour, I noticed my friend, Enna, in her own dance. Tall and strong, she moved gracefully through the space, seeming totally at ease. I could hear her sandals slapping against the marble floor, the rhythm changing as she transitioned between walking, spinning, and staccato movements.

Enna looked up, and we made eye contact. In that brief exchange, we seemed to make a simultaneous decision: *Let's move together.*

As we danced closer to one another, I realized I felt comfortable. Enna had been my roommate during the workshop, and we had supported each other during weak, vulnerable moments. I had cared for her when she had had a fever, and she had watched over me when the pollution of the city had left me nauseated and weak. Now, here we both were, strong and recovered. I sensed that my friendship with Enna had a solid foundation of mutual honor, trust, and respect. Out of everyone, she was the person with whom I would be most comfortable practicing inter-independence.

Taking a breath, I set an intention: I would stay committed to my full self-expression. I would not collapse or forego my authentic desires when dancing with Enna. As we began to interact, I noticed how her movements impacted my inner experience. Even when it felt uncomfortable, I continued to honor my commitment. Sometimes, this meant slowing down when Enna sped up. Other times, it meant stepping back to take more space.

At one point, Enna came very close to me, and I felt my body constrict. Typically, this would have started an internal debate: Should I suffer through my discomfort to show I welcomed her expression? Or should I move away at the risk of offending her and having her leave? Today, however, my inner dialogue was different.

This is an important moment, I told myself. *You cannot ignore your needs in order to please others. You have to take care of yourself, even if that means someone doesn't like what you're doing and wants to move on.*

Reminding myself of the strong relationship I'd built with Enna, I allowed myself to step back. As I moved away, the tension in my body dissolved. I once again felt centered. I watched for Enna's reaction. She stayed nearby, engaged with her own movement and available for more interaction.

My fear transformed into curiosity as this crucial moment opened a new inquiry. As Enna moved, which new position would allow me to maintain a sense of both partnership and comfortable internal spaciousness? Could I hold onto that feeling in each and every changing moment? What would it be like to test Enna's boundaries, trusting that if I got too close, she would take care of herself?

As I began to explore these questions, the dance with Enna became a playful interaction. We each moved at our own pace, giving one another enough time to recalibrate and find a sense of grounded presence. Every moment felt complete in itself, and I savored both my inner experience and the one I was sharing with Enna. I noticed I was not attached to our interaction and had no expectation or need for it to continue. In honoring myself, I was able to keep a healthy sense of perspective.

Eventually, Enna moved away. I didn't feel left behind, ignored, or unseen. I felt grateful for what we had created, and no need to hold onto it.

Knowing how inter-independence felt meant I now had a touchstone. Whether I was practicing Amerta Movement or navigating a new relationship, I could look to this memory in the pendopo as an example of how to honor my self-expression in a way that led to healthy, sustainable interactions.

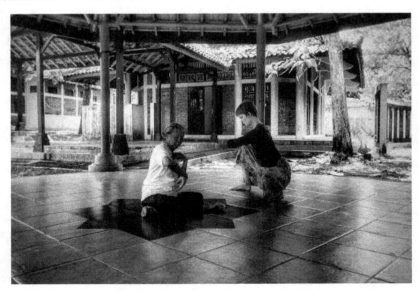

The author (right) practicing beside Prapto in the Wisma Seni
pendopo in Solo, Java, April 2017
Photo credit: Anonymous

***

Over the next 12 days, as Prapto's workshop traveled to the sacred sites of Candi Sukuh on Mount Lawu, the Parangtritis coast, Candi Borobudur, and Candi Boko, I continued to find richness in the practice of inter-independence. It was an incredible journey, but as my time in Java came to an end, I was ready to return home. My prior travels through India, Thailand, and Indonesia had taken a toll on my health due to environmental toxicity. While I did have to spend the next several months recovering, I never once regretted my time abroad.

What I learned from Prapto about inter-independence has become a part of my life. By practicing Amerta Movement, I have cultivated deep, mutually respectful relationships within a community of people who know and appreciate who I am, and I can express myself openly with my friends, parents, students, and even strangers without the shadow of fear that used to plague those interactions. I am confident that I have the right to be who I am, wherever I am.

On December 29, 2019, Prapto passed away at the age of 74. As I grieve this great loss, I feel even more grateful for what he taught me. I am inspired to apply principles from Amerta Movement in my workshops, with the hope that I can share some of the wisdom I received from Prapto.

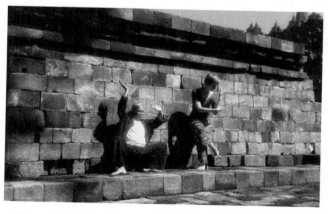

The author (right) practicing beside Prapto at
Borobudur Temple in Central Java, April 2017
Photo credit: Anonymous

Acknowledgements: Many thanks to Yana K.M., founder of Livingmyth.ru, for recommending I join Prapto's workshop and for connecting me with Diane Butler, PhD, in Bali. I am grateful for the spiritually and culturally enriching Awakening InterArts sessions Diane guided, and for her support in connecting me with Prapto, whom I honor as my mentor. As stated on the Padepokan Lemah Putih website, Prapto's Joged Amerta is "more than an approach to improvisation." Rather, it is "a practice cultivating an attitude towards life." Kind regards to Julie Nathanielsz, MFA, a 2016–2017 US Fulbright Scholar, for her talk "Place Making Body/Body Making Place," which boosted my confidence to travel to Java. A heartfelt thank-you goes out to my dear friend, Enna Kukkola, from Finland, for her emotional support during our shared experience in Java. I also dedicate this story in loving memory of Jordyn Ashley Newman, who inspired me to live fearlessly and to follow my inner calling without delay.

Recommended resources:

Amerta Movers. (n.d.). Retrieved July 06, 2020, from http://www.amertamovers.wordpress.com/

Butler, D. (n.d.). Awakening InterArts Workshops. Retrieved July 06, 2020, from https://www.facebook.com/AwakeningInterArtsworkshops

Living Myth. (n.d.). Retrieved July 06, 2020, from http://livingmyth.ru/

Padepokan Lemah Putih. (n.d.). Retrieved July 06, 2020, from http://www.lemahputih.com/

THE WEIGHT OF THE RAIN

Helen Styring Tocci

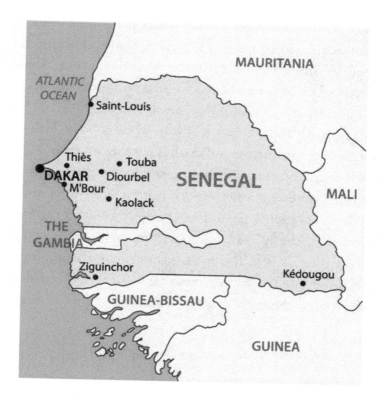

About the author: Helen Styring Tocci is a New York City-based teaching artist, musician, choreographer, and director, as well as the co-founder of the Varoom Group Dance Collective. For 20 years, she has focused on supporting people of all ages as they explore their creativity and discover the innate strength and wisdom that lives in every body. Helen is a certified yoga instructor and teaches workshops nationally in Circus Yoga, contact improvisation, and fusion partner dance. Helen has received artist grants from the Field and the Brooklyn Arts Exchange, and was recently awarded the Dani Nikas Excellence in Teaching Award for her work with New York City youth. She holds BAs in dance performance/composition and religious studies from Connecticut College. Read more about Helen and her projects at www.helenstyringtocci.com.

It began with the waiting... waiting for the rain. The cloud was just a smudge on the horizon when I first arrived at my host family's home in Sédhiou, Senegal. It had grown steadily closer as the days went by, its eventual arrival as sure as my love for this newfound home, the weight of my breasts against my chest, and the abiding beat of my heart.

This waiting was some of the sweetest time I've known. Sometimes we chatted, Pape and I: he would tease me in his quickly improving English, or I would shyly practice my French. Perched on the edge of the rickety wooden porch, the substantial curve of my hip pressed against his leanness, we sat. His legs swung freely, while mine stayed tucked underneath me, our fingers threaded lightly together, with our palms held apart to avoid the heat.

Sometimes we drank the sweet, dark ataya tea (as dark as the night sky in this rural village) that was traditionally served in three rounds. The first round was a bite on the tongue from the strong tannins in the fresh brew. Each round after was progressively tamer until we were simply sipping sugar water and giggling. Once in a while, my host sister, Nene, would silence us with a stern word.

"*Taisez-vous!* Be quiet, or you'll wake the little ones!" she would say. Her voice sounded serious, but when I caught her eye, her face betrayed her. She could not help but smile at our delight.

Sometimes Pape and I were the calm, watchful eye at the center of a whirlwind, as children and chickens kicked up clouds of dust that rose in spirals around us. We reveled in their antics and the simple joy of being alive and together in this place—two strangers from opposite sides of the world, who were now like family.

At other times, we sat in silence, simply watching the huge, ever-changing cloud grow inexorably closer. It felt like years we had been waiting, sitting hand in hand in the dirt yard, under the mango tree. By the end of my stay, the cloud was luminous and pink and very, very close: so close it tinted the hot, humid air with a rosy glow. It loomed over us, and we had to lie on our backs in the dirt yard to take it all in. I lay in its shadow, my head resting comfortably against Pape's, my body released fully into the ground, and my breathing soft and shallow.

Somehow, I was both perfectly content to be where I was and longing for the waiting to end.

***

I had arrived in Senegal months earlier, eager to start my trip with Intercultural Dimensions, a nonprofit company that promotes cross-cultural awareness through travel, community service, and workshops. My fellow participants and I were intent on learning as much as we could about Senegalese culture. We flew into the capital city of Dakar, the westernmost tip of a peninsula that extends from the mainland into the Atlantic Ocean. We then traveled along the lush green coast, taking in the incredible beauty of golden sands backed by low cliffs. Along the way, we passed colorful houses crafted from stone, shell, and driftwood.

From there, we turned inland and made our way across the Gambian border toward the remote jungle villages of southern Senegal. During our four weeks of travel, we would visit cultural art centers, hospitals, and schools throughout the country. Everywhere – *everywhere* – we were greeted by dancing. Although I had danced my whole life, I had never experienced dance the way I had in Senegal.

***

I discovered dance in an austere, but beautiful, church hall in northern Vermont that served as a ballet studio. When I would stand at the bar with my peers, my curves looked like strange, fecund flowers among the slender, willowy bodies of the other ballerinas. Growing up in the 80s, when calorie counting and Jane Fonda workouts were all the rage, I was taught my weight was a problem. It was something to be highly managed and generally ashamed of. My middle school friends giggled when I told them I was studying ballet, eyeing the wideness of my newly acquired hips and heavy, round breasts.

I felt stifled by the rigidity of the ballet technique I was learning, like it was a dress that covered too much of me and fit a bit too tightly. In our small-town ballet shows, I was always given the part of the wicked witch or the rat queen, as if my weight somehow made me evil. While I relished the overt theatricality and athleticism of these roles, deep down I yearned for the freedom of the sublime sugar plum fairy who flitted across the stage, floating above it all in ethereal splendor.

Despite ballet's uneasy fit, I still felt beautiful when I was dancing. I found solace in the studio, where I could connect to my body, feel the power in my muscles, and tune into the impulses that arose in me. I wasn't yet sure what to do with these inclinations, for my strict ballet training did not allow me to embrace them.

Later, I found ways to express myself more freely. I danced with newfound independence and agency as I learned the joys of modern dance in the studios of my liberal arts college. Even in this more expansive environment, however, I spent years trying to look and be like the slender dancers I admired, rather than embracing my own shape. I did my best to dance like them, fighting how I instinctively wanted to move and shunning my natural body size, as well as the momentum and connection to the earth that my weight affords.

***

In Senegal, I quickly discovered that people's relationship to dance was different.

When we arrived at a school outside of Dakar early in my trip, we were greeted by a crowd of joyful, dancing children. Drummers appeared, and a performance of welcome began. Sometimes, the children danced in unison, jumping athletically and performing complicated, rhythmic Wolof steps typical of the northern region of Senegal. Other times, they surrounded us and improvised to the drums with abandon. Their hands reached toward us in welcome, and their smiles let us know how happy they were to share this time with us.

Wherever we went, everyone danced. Dance was a way to celebrate being alive and together in community. People danced to welcome new visitors, to celebrate important events, or simply because they were happy. People danced whether they were curvy, angular, or somewhere in between.

While there were professional dance companies in Senegal, such as the Senegalese National Ballet, dance was not restricted to those with formal training. Everyone danced, not just those with experience and the right bodies. Everyone.

Watching the children at the school dance that day, I was delighted... until they asked me to join in.

"Dance for us!" the children cried, skipping around me with bright, expectant faces.

"I'm shy," I told them hesitantly in my broken French.

The truth, however, was that I wasn't sure how to join them. How could I dance if I didn't know the steps or if the performance wasn't planned? What would they think of me if I did it wrong? What if my dance wasn't good enough? My body tightened into knots as the hopeful expressions on their shining faces faded into looks of confusion.

"Why would you be shy to dance?" they asked, as if dancing for others were as simple as shaking hands or as automatic as breathing.

I tried to explain how it was back home. I'd always thought of dancing as something to be practiced, painstakingly labored over, perfected, edited, and critiqued. Only then could you share your dance with others. But no matter what I said, the children persisted. They simply wanted to dance with me!

Eventually, out of respect for me as their guest, they stopped asking.

This pattern would continue at every stop on our itinerary. There would be a joyful dance of welcome, my bashful rebuff and finally our Senegalese hosts' amiable – but perplexed – acceptance. These experiences always left me unsatisfied. Although I was scared to explore this raw, authentic relationship to dance, I also deeply longed for the level of freedom I saw in the dancers in Senegal. I wanted to be able to dance without knowing which step was next, to have my movement be an expression of my emotions, to be in the present moment with my body and its connection to the world, and to allow the music and the energy of those around me to choose how the dance unfolded. I felt these things were possible, but I had no idea how to begin.

As we continued to travel through the country, my desire to accept these invitations grew. Then, after one challenging night in a tiny village in the Casamance region, things changed.

We were deep in the jungle, where the only light that distracted us from the brilliant canopy of stars was from the communal cooking fires. It had taken us many hours to reach this remote community, and I arrived feeling ill. The long day bumping along in the back of the Jeep had left me weak and woozy, and a month of daily tea ceremonies had taken a toll on my digestion. I felt dizzy, and my stomach ached with constipation.

We finally arrived at the entrance of the village, where the local chief and his wife greeted us. I listened to their introductions and pleasantries through a feverish haze, and tried to smile and nod respectfully as they told us about the dancing and drumming they had planned for our evenings. Just when they were introducing us to the goat they would be slaughtering for a feast in our honor, I fainted.

I spent that night curled in a ball on the dirt in the chief's garden, my head over the deep hole that served as a latrine. The chief's wife stayed with me, holding my hair, rubbing my back, and whispering soothing words in my ear. While I couldn't understand what she was saying, her presence comforted me. I was deeply touched by her care, especially since we had just met. By morning, I was emptied out and weak, but clear headed. The chief greeted me as his wife helped me back into their thatched-roof home.

"Now," he said in French, folding my small hand in between his two larger ones, "you are one of us, my dear." It seemed he considered the generosity and kindness his wife had bestowed upon me as a way to welcome me into his family.

He smiled down at me, as if I hadn't just kept his wife up all night, weren't covered in sweat and dirt, and didn't smell to high hell. His smile was a blessing.

Something shifted in me that morning. Perhaps it was the chief and his wife's support, or perhaps throwing up publicly all night had dissolved my inhibitions. Either way, I felt different. Their generous acceptance of me, even when I was at my worst, had unlocked an entirely new sense of safety and freedom.

That night, the whole village gathered in a circle around a blazing bonfire. Drummers played as everyone took their turn coming to the center and sharing their dance. Previously, I would have watched this with dread, knowing someone would try to draw me into the circle to perform. This night, however, I did not worry. I trusted that their invitation was not a challenge or an opportunity for them to judge, but for me to be a part of the community, to share myself.

Growing up, I'd learned that I needed to be good at something or not do it at all. But here, these ideals of perfectionism – like making the ideal first impression – didn't seem to matter. In this community, allowing myself to be vulnerable seemed to deepen the relationship with those around me, rather than incite judgement.

As I watched the others dance that night, I felt my excitement rising.

"Be with us!" their rhythmic stamping seemed to say.

"Show us who you are!" their undulating bodies sang.

A desire to dance ebbed and flowed within me. It would grow as I became inspired by their joyful self-expression and the communal energy, only to dissolve as I worried about getting the steps right. Though my self-consciousness had not entirely disappeared, that night, when my new friends' eyes turned towards me, my fear did not stop me. I entered the circle of firelight.

My dance was far from perfect. As the drummers played, I improvised some ballet, stringing together movements learned over a decade of sweat, patience, and strict practice. My pointed toes and erect posture stood in stark contrast to the bent knees, athletic bearing, and sinuously strong movements of the Senegalese dancers.

Even so, they were delighted that I had joined them. They clapped their hands, and I felt encouraged by their smiles. They giggled, but they weren't being mean or teasing. My audience was genuinely charmed by my movements, chuckling like you would at a child's adorable antics. It did seem, however, like they were also waiting for something else—some other way I could move that they knew was possible, but that I couldn't yet imagine.

The next morning, I was sad to leave the village, but also extremely excited for the next stage of my journey. Sédiou, a town nestled in a curve of the great Casamance River, was the last stop on our tour and the place where I would say goodbye to the rest of my travel companions. I'd elected to extend my study of Senegalese music and dance through a homestay with Alioune Diedhiou, a dear friend of the organizers of Intercultural Dimensions who had invited me to live with his family for several months. This way, I could work with local dancers and drummers, improving my skills with consistent teachers and immersing myself in the arts, music, and dance of a local community.

When I arrived at the Diedhiou compound, it was dinnertime, and the whole family gathered to welcome me. Diedhiou's wife, Fatou Dieme, greeted me with a quiet confidence, her voice soft but steady. She introduced me to their eight children in order of age: there was Omar, the eldest; Ibou; Seynebou; Laila; and sparkly-eyed Nene, who greeted me with a mischievous wink. I knew in that moment that Nene and I would be friends. Next came Amy, Samba, and Bouly, the youngest, who toddled, giggling, right into my arms.

Only after I'd met all the children did I meet Pape, a young man who was boarding with the family. I immediately loved his huge smile and the carefree way he cocked his head as he waved his hello. He greeted me enthusiastically, and I shyly said hello.

Pape would soon become one of my closest friends. He could always be counted on for a joke when I was feeling down, or to challenge me to step into an adventure. Nearly every day, he would surprise me with some little gift: a ripe mango he had harvested from the top of a tree, a bird's nest he'd found hidden in the back garden, a quirky (and usually slightly naughty) story explaining something about Senegalese culture, or a new rhythm he had learned to play on the djembe. He said he loved to see me smile, and he often inspired me to do so. His freedom and vibrant joy delighted me!

As I sat down for my first meal with the family, the cloud was only a promise on the horizon, its glorious colors and the beauty of its luscious curves yet to be discovered. It sat in the distance, expectant like a full-belly breath just waiting to be released. The table was set under the mango tree in the dusty courtyard, its vibrant leaves and fecund fruit a striking contrast to the scorched brown earth. Even in the dry season, Fatou and Nene had managed to make the compound homey with intricately patterned *boubous* (typical Senegalese tunics) hanging from the drying line, and bright batiked cloths bringing color and life to the windows and tables.

Over the next few days, the Diedhiou family invited me fully into their life, integrating me into their routines and allowing me to ask any question in my slowly improving French. They spent hours familiarizing me with the customs of their town: how to draw water from the well for my bucket bath, prepare different Senegalese delicacies, and respectfully greet others, for traditional greetings are a huge part of Senegalese social customs.

When Nene and I would make our way to the market, we would stop at least ten times to say hello to neighbors and friends.

"*I be heera to?* (Are you in peace?)" Nene would ask a group of women in brightly colored *boubous* (traditional, lightweight garments), speaking in Mandinka.

"*Heera doroŋ* (Peace only)," they would reply.

"*Kori tana nteŋ?* (You have no harm?)"

"*Tana nteŋ.* (No harm.)"

"*Suukononkoolu lee?* (How is everyone in your family?)"

"*I bee be jee.* (They are there.)"

On and on the greetings would go over a prolonged handshake. In Sédiou, nothing was ever done in a hurry. With more than 10 different languages spoken in the town alone, learning how to greet our neighbors was quite a task. Getting to the market that was located a five-minute walk from our house was often a journey that took the bulk of the morning. In Sédiou, people seemed to prioritize connection over anything else, and took their time with things they felt were important. I was in awe of the care that the townsfolk displayed for each other and the freedom they gave themselves to follow their own rhythms.

All the members of Diedhiou's family contributed to the household. Visiting the market was just one of Nene's many daily tasks. I was surprised by how much responsibility the young women assumed. At 16, Nene was considered a full-fledged woman in Senegalese society and expected to spend the day working in the home. She, along with Fatou and the other teenage girls, were in charge of cooking, cleaning the compound, and looking after the younger children. She was quite a bit younger than I was, but felt like a friend. We giggled over village gossip while she taught me the proper way to care for a Senegalese home. I deeply admired Nene's skill and competence, and felt in awe of the incredible responsibility she shouldered at such a young age.

The men of the family spent their time working the land. Peanuts and millet were a primary source of income for the family and also featured prominently in our meals. Since it was the dry season, and the Casamance was in the midst of a drought, the men were working especially hard to make ends meet. Every day, they would leave the village to work the fields, and Pape would go with them. He would trail behind despite Diedhiou's calls to keep up, making me laugh with a silly walking dance, for he knew I was sad when he left. The men would return from their labors in the evening to a home expertly cared for by the women of the family.

At mealtimes, we would gather around a large communal platter of rice or millet. The grain was always covered in sauce and layered with vegetables, as well as chicken or fish. My favorite meal was *Yassa poisson*, a Senegalese delicacy of fish smothered in lemon, garlic, and mustard sauce.

As we ate, Diedhiou would flick the choicest pieces of fish or meat to my portion of the platter with his long, thin fingers. It was often more than I could ever eat. Over time, we developed a playful game, flicking the extra meat back and forth across the platter. This delighted the youngsters, who giggled at the indignity of grownups playing with their food. Inevitably, Pape would end up with any leftovers, for he had a fast-growing teenage body—and also the quickest hands.

While these moments made me feel at home, they also represented my unusual standing in the family. I existed in a liminal space: too grown up to be a child, but too culturally different to contribute to my family as a typical adult. I had the body of a woman, but none of the responsibilities that Senegalese women acquire at a much younger age. And, as a foreign guest, I was often treated like a man: served first at the table and given consideration in any discussion.

In some ways, living this way was incredibly freeing. I could explore and try new things without any fear of judgment. People generally regarded my actions as strange, but harmless and amusing. In other ways, however, it was lonely. I never felt fully a part of any group. Over the coming weeks, as my Senegalese family grew closer and closer to my heart, I carried this awareness of separateness with me, bittersweet and necessary.

Some days, being a woman-child with only basic French skills felt strange, tiring, and overwhelming. I never completely grasped anything, nor was I ever fully understood by those around me. I constantly ached for my family, far away in the States. Then, in the 90s, no one in the village had a phone, and letters were the only way for me to communicate with those at home.

The Diedhiou family had given me my own room, an incredible luxury in a space that housed more than a dozen people. On the days when the loneliness was most acute, I would curl up on my bed, pull out my battery-powered Walkman, and try not to feel guilty about the indulgence of this space and quiet. The mosquito net reduced the world outside to a soft blur, and for a moment, the music transported me home.

I was profoundly uncomfortable in this in-between space, holding so many opposites and stretching the confines of who I thought I was, but there was also freedom here. And as I felt the support and love more and more strongly from Pape, Nene, and the community of friends I had made, this uneasy, in-between space became a place where I could explore who I was and the possibility of who I could become.

After I had rested in my room for a while, one of the babies would peek into the room giggling, or there'd be a kerfuffle in the yard as Pape stalked a chicken for dinner, or I'd hear the chatter of a neighbor stopping by for a visit. When I felt ready, I would rejoin the family, for they missed me when I was gone. I would make my way quietly to the porch, watch the sunset's glow behind the ever-growing cloud, and wonder when the rains would come.

***

My days in Sédiou took on an easy pattern as I began my studies in music and dance. Mornings were spent at the home of Monsieur Mané, a master musician descended from a long line of musicians. He was charged with teaching me to play the *balafon*, an ancient West African gourd-resonating xylophone typically made with a bamboo frame and wooden keys.

Diedhiou walked me to M. Mané's home for my first lesson. He introduced me to my new teacher, who silently took my hand and shook it gently and thoughtfully. M. Mané's face, filled with lines, looked like carved obsidian. He was stoic as he silently handed me a hatchet and led me to a corner of his yard.

I was confused. Why was he giving me a hatchet instead of mallets to play the balafon? And where were the instruments? I soon figured out (for I heard not a word from M. Mané, nor would I until many days later) that we would be crafting my balafon from a fallen tree and gourds harvested from his garden.

For several weeks we worked tirelessly, cutting out the rough key shapes with hatchets, sanding the wood into smooth-as-silk planks, and binding these planks together into a rough xylophone shape. We then dried the gourds and tied them under the wooden planks, ready to capture the sound and provide resonance. Only then did we begin the long, painstaking process of sanding the wooden keys to tune them.

After a month, my instrument was finally ready. With my heart beating excitedly, I sat down across from M. Mané, the balafon stretched between us like a rope bridge over a deep ravine. In my sweaty hands, I held the mallets we had carved from wood scraps and crowned with rubber-band balls. They were similar to the ones M. Mané held: the ones he had just used to play the most complex and beautiful music I had ever heard. Now, he was attempting to break down what each hand must do to replicate the song.

M. Mané was teaching me a polyrhythm, the simultaneous combination of contrasting rhythms that each have a different beat subdivision. The tension and release found in polyrhythms make them incredibly danceable—and very different from the typical four-on-the-floor pattern that I had grown accustomed to in the States.

I practiced each hand's rhythm religiously until I could play with my eyes closed. Hard as I tried, however, I couldn't play the two sides together. The two rhythms seemed so completely unique, each entirely unrelated to the other. As I tried for perhaps the 20th time to master the polyrhythm, a low, sharp *humph* of annoyance rumbled from M. Mané's lips. He got to his feet and left the pavilion. It was the first noise I'd ever heard M. Mané make... and it was not the words of encouragement I'd hoped for.

My afternoon dance lessons were progressing slightly better. I was learning from Fatou Sula Tamba, a small, stout woman with a mischievous smile and seemingly boundless energy who was well known as the best dancer in town. We established an immediate connection and method of working together. She would dance, and I would follow behind her, trying to copy whichever step she decided it was time for me to learn.

When we first started, I had expected to learn the flashy moves of the Senegalese dances I had seen performed in the States, most of which came from the northern Wolof tradition. Fatou Sula Tamba, however, wanted to teach me the much more subtle dances of the Balante people of southern Senegal. These dances were more focused on nuanced rhythms in the body and small, syncopated steps.

For days and days, I followed Fatou Sula Tamba around the dusty yard, trying my hardest to capture the beautiful, rhythmic patterns that flowed so seamlessly through her form. The polyrhythms, I was discovering, were not just in the music. They were also in the dance! Fatou Sula Tamba's body was so different from the thin dancers' bodies I had been raised to emulate, and her dancing was indescribably beautiful to me. I had never worked with a dancer whose curves matched or exceeded my own. As I watched her, I noticed something was missing in my own movement. Much like with the balafon, I had learned what each part of my body was supposed to be doing, but I couldn't feel how it all came together.

And then one day, I did. Two hours into a rehearsal inside my teacher's home, I was tired and hungry. Distracted by my discomfort, I had stopped thinking so hard about how my various body parts should move. I was no longer trying to emulate Fatou Sula Tamba. In fact, I wasn't even watching her, but simply dancing and admiring how the light streaming through the open doorway made the dust sparkle. I closed my eyes and felt the warmth of the sun on my chest and belly, which relaxed in response to my soft attention. Suddenly, there it was: the polyrhythm. I felt it as a continuous waterfall moving through my shoulder blades, flowing into my chest, spiraling around my ribs, undulating through my hips, and finally falling through my legs to be picked up again by my feet. My entire body moved in concert, a whole orchestra in one organism.

I danced blissfully with my eyes closed, the sun shining in on me, for a long time. If I focused on just one part of my body, everything fell apart. But if I simply allowed myself to trust the weight of my body, feel my connection with the ground, and allow the rhythm of the music to move me, the polyrhythm persisted.

When I finally opened my eyes, I saw that Fatou Sula Tamba had turned around and was watching me. The beginnings of a smile crinkled her eyes.

"Come," she said. "Let's get some food."

The next morning, I arrived early at M. Mané's house. By the time he made his way to the pavilion with his steaming cup of tea, I already had my balafon ready, mallets in hand. He eyed me silently before sitting down and playing the rhythm we had worked on for days. This time, I didn't keep my eyes glued to his hands, trying desperately to make sense of the disparate parts. I closed my eyes and let the music wash over me. Instead of holding so tightly to each separate rhythm, I tried to feel the song as a whole. When M. Mané finished, I picked up my mallets and played. While the music faltered at times, and was much slower than M. Mané's rhythm, I was playing his song. When I finished, I laid down the mallets and looked up. M. Mané was smiling.

"Yoooooo..." he said in his deep, raspy voice. This was the first and last time I would hear him speak. The sound of his approval reverberated through my whole body. It was as warm as the sunlight.

I had plenty of time to practice this newfound sense of rhythm, for my host brothers and sisters loved to go out at night to the town's many discotheques. In Sédhiou, these were simply rooms that were large enough to fit many sweaty bodies in motion, and that possessed sufficient electricity for a sound system and an aspiring DJ. There, surrounded by Nene, Pape, and my other host siblings, I would dance with a newfound freedom.

One night, feeling beautifully relaxed after so much dancing, we walked home together just as the sky was beginning to lighten, a golden glow on the horizon and the persistent stars still twinkling high above our heads. We went slowly, our bodies spent from the night's madness. I was surrounded by my family, our pinkies linked, for it was far too hot for any more contact than that.

In the presence of their acceptance, I had found the space to release my self-consciousness and surrender to the joy of dancing. Feeling so connected to these people I loved, I was more comfortable in my body than ever before. Around us, the village was starting to come alive. I heard a rooster crow, a baby's cry, birds calling good morning, and the occasional rustle of palm leaves above as an animal shot past us in pursuit of breakfast. The smell of freshly baked French bread stopped us in our tracks. As we stood there, enjoying the enticing aroma and the sounds of the waking world around us, the baker poked his head out and sent us on our way with a treat, fresh from the oven. It burned our fingers, but we ate it greedily anyway—high on life, dancing, and the joy of unexpected gifts.

***

The next time the town gathered to dance (as they regularly did), I eagerly joined in the crowd. I watched as dancers of all shapes and sizes shimmied, jumped, and twirled with abandon. When they gestured for me to join, I did so with an open heart and a free mind. I danced not for a teacher in a class or for an anonymous audience, but as an offering for my community. I was dancing to be seen, to represent my belonging, and to celebrate my body and its connection to the earth. I danced the truth of the gravity in my bones, the rushing of my blood, the beautiful weight of my muscles, and the joy rising in my heart. The polyrhythms flowed through me, and I allowed those present to see me in my fullness. My freedom gave them joy. This time, when I finished dancing and looked up, I saw something new on their faces: respect.

I walked home that evening by myself under the wide canopy of stars, feeling the expansiveness of the sky reflected inside of me. With the release of all those years of struggle to make my body conform to what others deemed acceptable, there was suddenly so much space for who I actually wanted to be. I reveled in my newfound agency to express myself, and a joy and deep appreciation for my weight. My shape made my offering solely my own. I'm one of the strongest, most nimble dancers I know. If I had a skinny body, I wouldn't have my dance—my self-expression articulated through my distinct shape.

That day, I found the philosophy I now share with my students: Our bodies are our own unique instrument, and each instrument has a special purpose. This is what brings beauty to the world. We don't all have the same gift, and we don't all make the same offering. Our job, contrary to so much of what we are told, is not to judge what we've been given. Instead, we must find what we are meant to express, and to use our instrument to do so as fully as possible.

***

It was just a few days before Diedhiou would take me on the 12-hour bus trip through the Casamance, across The Gambia, and along the coast back to Dakar, where I would board a plane for the flight back to the United States.

The big cloud, dark and low in the sky and heavy with rain, was looming overhead. Pape, Nene, and I sat in the shade of the mango tree, too hot to even speak. I was overwhelmed by my imminent departure, and I felt the preciousness of every moment in this place and with these beloved people.

But this time, when I felt overwhelmed, I did not hide away. I went to my room, brought out my Walkman, and turned the headphones outward. With our sweaty foreheads pressed together, I shared those precious bits of my home and heart with Pape and Nene. As Tracy Chapman's voice, with all its caramel richness, floated into the air around us, I tried my best to translate "The Promise" into French for Pape. Pape, in turn, translated from French to Diola for Nene.

As Tracy sang of faith, hope, and the abiding ties of love, big tears began to slide down Nene's cheeks. I knew she understood. Although we might never see each other again, they would always hold a place in my heart. I stopped translating, and we just sat together, the music holding us with its sweetness and sorrow. I decided my Walkman and the music would stay behind with them when I left.

***

I can't remember exactly what I was doing when the big cloud opened and finally released the weight of the rain. Perhaps Pape and I were resting, stretched out in the dirt under the mango tree as we often were in the afternoon when the air was thick and close, our shoulders touching and eyes nearly closed. Maybe he had climbed up the tree to pick a mango for us to share with the children gathered around, eagerly awaiting pieces of the luscious fruit. I could have been sitting with Nene in the outdoor kitchen, going over the finer nuances of fish preparation. I might have been keeping her company in the shade of the porch as she ironed clothes and we giggled over some village gossip, Bouly squirming in my arms as I attempted to rock him to sleep. Or perhaps the whole family had gathered in the yard, as they often did, enjoying the sunset as it painted its magnificent colors across the huge cloud that had taken over the sky.

What I do remember is the sound of the raindrops. Everything was silent except for the *slap, slap, slap* of the water hitting the parched earth. It was as if time had stopped.

Then there was an explosion of sound. The adults—and even stoic Diedhiou!—jumped to their feet, hugged each other, and joyfully bounded onto the covered porch. Everyone was smiling, and we heaved a collective sigh of deep relief and contentment. For the adults, the coming of the rain meant the lands that were their livelihood would be nourished, their family fed, and the village protected.

The children were not thinking about the future, but instinctively knew the joy of release. They ran straight out into the rain to dance, welcoming it with as much delight as the Senegalese had shown when welcoming me to their country those many months ago. To the surprise and amazement of the adults, I threw on my bathing suit and ran to join the kids. We jumped and splashed and twirled through the rivers of mud, giggling as we held hands and tried to catch raindrops on our tongues. In that moment, I was the freest I had ever been in my body. I felt the years of conditioning, criticism, and harsh judgment about how I should look sliding off my shoulders with the raindrops. I was left feeling simultaneously so light and so beautifully heavy.

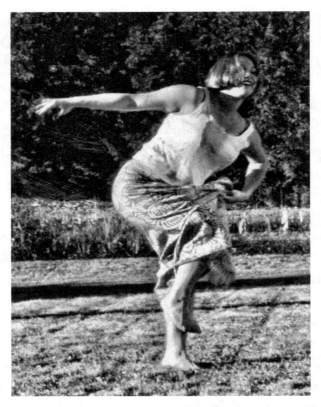

The author dances at her family's home in Vermont just after
returning from Senegal in August 1998
Photo credit: Greg Tocci

Dedication: This story is dedicated to Alioune, Nene, Pape, and the entire Diedhiou family, as well as to M. Malang Mané and Fatou Sula Tamba. I am humbled by and deeply grateful for the incredible generosity, openness, and love with which you welcomed me into your homes and shared your wisdom. Although time and space has long separated us, know that you are forever in my heart.

Recommended resources:

The music of Baba Maal
Waato Siita. (n.d.). Retrieved July 08, 2020, from http://waatosiita.com/

COURAGE

Megan Taylor Morrison

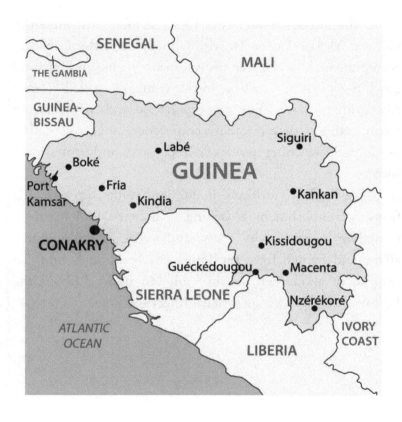

About the author: In January 2015, a year after returning from Guinea, Megan Taylor Morrison finally took the leap into entrepreneurship. Her first two ventures – a life and business coaching practice, and a travel company called Dance Adventures – have since supported thousands of people in reconnecting to their creativity, confidence, and sense of play, as well as in reaching new levels of personal and professional success.

Meg holds a certificate in life and leadership coaching from Accomplishment Coaching, a master's in journalism from Northwestern University, and a BA in international affairs and French from the University of Puget Sound. To read more about her, see her full bio under "About the Editors," or visit www.megantaylormorrison.com.

Inside the concrete gymnasium, the air was hot and damp. Dust-speckled sunshine filtered into the space through small, paneless windows high up on the walls, creating diluted spotlights on the floor. A gaggle of wide-eyed children gathered around a large, crumbling hole in the cinder block structure: the doorway to this dim, austere space. The kids giggled as they arranged themselves in the best viewing position, with the taller ones in back.

My fellow travelers and I sat against the wall of this *maison de jeunesse* (youth center), one of many similar structures sprinkled throughout Guinea's capital, Conakry. Everyone here was waiting expectantly for the rehearsal of one of the city's talented *ballets* (performance groups), Ballet Matambe, to begin.

"These buildings serve as community hubs," said Sarah Lee Parker, one of the leaders of our artistic immersion program. "Their most common use is as a practice space."

"I love that places like this are so accessible," I responded, thinking back to how challenging it had been to find affordable practice spots in the US cities I'd called home.

"Well, it's not that clear cut," Sarah Lee replied. "The maisons de jeunesse are typically booked morning to night, and they often have waiting lists. This is a big topic of conversation right now between the artistic community and local politicians. There's a need for much more space."

I nodded, appreciating the clarification. Since I'd arrived, I'd learned a lot from Sarah Lee, our other hosts, and – most of all – my Guinean teachers about what it meant to be a professional artist in Conakry. Although I'd had similar discussions with dancers and musicians in the United States and abroad, the magnitude of challenges that creatives faced here felt unique. Over and over, I had found myself humbled by their quiet perseverance.

Deep in thought, I looked out the door of the maison de jeunesse. The sky was clear, and I could hear the sound of drumming on the breeze. Somewhere in the distance, perhaps in another building like this one, musicians were playing rhythms loved by Guineans for hundreds of years.

***

Nine months earlier, Sarah Lee had told me about the opportunity to visit Guinea.

"If you want to train with dedicated, insanely talented West African dancers and drummers, you need to come," she said.

While I'd had the chance to take classes from West African artists in the United States – including Etienne Cakpo, who had moved to the Pacific Northwest from Benin, and Youssouf Koumbassa, who taught at dance camps around the country – I wanted to take my education further. I believed that in order to be a conscious and respectful participant in West African Dance, it was important to study the history of the dances, see the parts of Guinea where certain traditions had originated, and better understand how this living, breathing art form was evolving. While I knew I could never fully grasp the cultural context of Guinean arts as a white American, I would do my best to learn as much as possible.

There was another reason I wanted to go: the trip had come at a time when I was struggling to find the courage to leave my full-time desk job and start down the path of artistic entrepreneurship. The idea of spending three full weeks with professional artists felt indescribably nourishing, and I imagined that I would find solace and inspiration in our conversations about their experiences.

The immersion program would be co-hosted by Mamady Mansare (a former member of Les Ballets Africains, one of the best known West African performance groups in the world and the first company of its kind to operate internationally) and his relatives. We would stay at the Mansare family compound, where we would also take singing, dancing, and drumming classes each day with members of Les Ballets Africains and other local dance groups. Sarah Lee, an instructor in West African dance at the University of Washington and the founder of One World Dance & Drum, would be there to help coordinate the trip.

282

At night, we would have free time to hang out with the artists, practice what we'd learned, or spend time in the neighborhood with our hosts. Without a local cell phone or a way to connect to the internet, I knew little would distract me from being present with the learning, community, and questions about my future.

***

From the very first day of our program, my fellow travelers and I had jumped on any opportunity to get to know the local performers better. Thus, we had eagerly agreed when Sarah Lee and Mamady had offered to take us to this rehearsal.

With the loud crack of a *djembe*, it began. The lead drummer pounded out the first beats, and a deafening chorus of *djembes* and *dunduns* answered. The sound of these West African instruments flooded the room. I covered my ears, and the music remained loud and clear.

The musicians, I realized, were playing a *kassa* rhythm, created by the Malinke ethnic group from the upper region of Guinea. I had learned to recognize this family of rhythms in my dance classes with Mamadama Bangoura, a principal dancer for Les Ballets Africains.

"Long ago, these songs and dances were done to encourage farmers as they worked out in the fields," she had told us. "Today, however, kassa is often performed by ballets across Conakry."

A dark mass swayed at the back of the room as forty dancers hidden in the shadows shifted into position. As the first performers emerged into the faint light, they formed a line that moved like a wave across the floor. Because of the intense heat, drops of sweat were already running down their faces.

The rhythm was fast – extremely fast – but the dancers were not daunted. They threw themselves into each step with full-bodied commitment. As they stretched dynamically into every movement, I heard shouts from the men and high-pitched shrieks of ecstasy from the women echo through the room. My eyes welled up with tears. Never before had I beheld such presence and power in movement, or this level of devotion to artistry.

***

Just hours before, when I had asked about the lifestyle of local artists, Mamadama had told me that many full-time, professional dancers and drummers worked night jobs at the airport to support themselves. After their shifts finished, they would walk eight miles to their practice space in the center of town. Furthermore, some only made enough money for one meal each day, and I couldn't imagine how much energy was required for these all-out rehearsals.

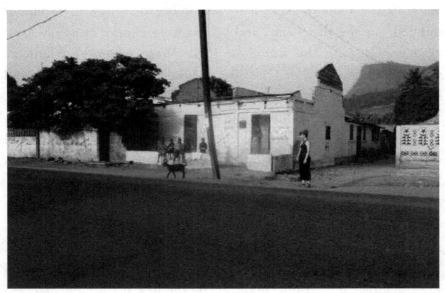

The author waits on the side of the road during a trip from Conakry to Kindia, Guinea Photo credit: Calico Goodrich

Despite challenges like these, Mamadama and the other artists I met kept our conversations focused on the positive. They loved the sense of community, the warmth of the people, and the amazing musicianship and dancing you could find in almost every corner of Guinea. They also often shared about how much they cherished their relationships with their friends and family, as well as their faith. Most of the people I met were Muslims, who heeded the prayer calls that echoed from the mosques five times each day.

Nevertheless, it was obvious that people were struggling with issues related to poverty and disease. Several times during my three-week stay, an artist would disappear for a day. When I would ask where they were, I would receive the answer in hushed tones: they'd gone across town or into the countryside to mourn the loss of a friend, parent, or teacher. The life expectancy in Guinea, I would later learn, was just 59 years for men and 60 for women, which is nearly 20 years shorter than that in the United States. This is due to many factors, including the prevalence of diseases such as malaria and tuberculosis.

The country's ongoing battle with polio was also apparent. One night, I had watched a jaw-dropping performance by a group called "Les Ambassadors de Personnes Handicapées de Guinée" (The Ambassadors for the Handicapped Persons of Guinea), who had all been crippled by the disease. These performers had moved with ferocious spirit, expressing themselves as well as or better than any able-bodied artist I'd met. No circumstance, it seemed, could get in the way of their dance. By the end of the show, my body was tingling. The air around me felt electric, like it was about to spark with possibility.

Watching these dancers, I wondered about the times I'd said something was "too hard" and had given up. When there was a challenge, did I give my all to overcome it? Did I even know what "giving my all" truly meant? As I made the transition into entrepreneurship, how could I totally and completely commit to my vocation, just as these artists committed to theirs?

***

Sitting in the maison de jeunesse that afternoon, I felt closer to full-out living and to death than ever before. As the rehearsal ended in a climax of room-shaking drumming, I wondered if living with that dichotomy was part of what made the performers this dynamic.

If so little were guaranteed in my own life, how would I live differently? I wondered. I imagined I'd make the most of each day—and, of course, each dance. I wouldn't save energy for later. Instead, I'd jump wholeheartedly into the present moment, making sure my movement would be part of my legacy.

Pondering this, I began reflecting on moments when I had seen my Guinean friends and teachers show up with what had seemed like inexhaustible big-heartedness, similar to what I'd just seen at this practice. During the six hours of classes I took with them each day, my teachers had patiently taught me the history of and moves to different rhythms from Guinea's four natural regions.

"There are Maritime Guinea, Middle Guinea, Upper Guinea, and Forested Guinea," Mamadama had told us. "We have a lot of diversity in our artistic traditions, given that Guinea's mountainous terrain historically kept each location fairly isolated. Today, however, artists here in Conakry do dances from all over the country."

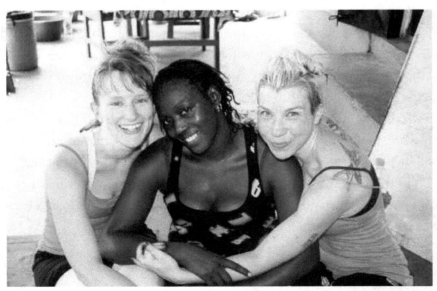

*From left, Megan Taylor Morrison, principal dancer of Les Ballets
Africains Mamadama Bangoura, and fellow dance adventurer Calico
Goodrich after a two-hour morning dance practice
Photo credit: Sarah Lee Parker*

It was an honor to study these dances and their accompanying songs and drum rhythms with Mamadama and the other dedicated, patient, talented instructors. I appreciated not only their vast knowledge, but also their encouragement to keep practicing in the face of various challenges. When I felt too tired to continue or my feet bled from dancing barefoot on the concrete, my teachers would look at me and smile.

"*Courage*, Megan!" they would say in French. And the drummers would play faster.

In this way, they lovingly pushed me past where I would otherwise have stopped, and urged me to keep going in the face of my own doubts and discomfort. I allowed them to guide me, knowing that learning to live with more fortitude would be invaluable as I worked toward my goals back at home.

***

Leaving the maison de jeunesse after the rehearsal, I was humbled once again. The performers I had just watched, as well as many other artists I'd met, embodied a level of courage I had never imagined. They embraced their identities as dancers or musicians, trained hard, and found a way to stay dedicated to their craft, no matter what happened.

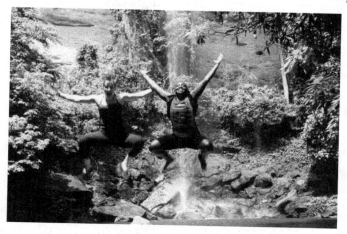

The author and Mamadama Bangoura in Kindia, Guinea
Photo credit: Sarah Lee Parker

As we walked along the dusty, unpaved streets of the neighborhood, I approached Sarah Lee.

"Meeting these artists and hearing their stories is really putting my fear in perspective," I told her. "If they have the courage to pursue their passion, who am I to deny mine? Even in my worst-case scenario, I can always make ends meet with a side job, move back in with my parents, or trade my car for public transit."

"Coming here helps us see the magnitude of our privilege and puts things in perspective," Sarah Lee replied, nodding. "My priorities have changed since my first visit. Money is much less important to me now, whereas community and doing work I believe in matter more."

For the duration of our journey back to the main road, I stayed quiet, noticing I was still terrified to leave my secure day job. I closed my eyes and took a few deep breaths, trying to picture the members of Ballet Matambe dancing full out. They had looked straight at me as they moved, and there had been no concern or self-doubt in their eyes. If I could live with half the power and intention represented in their dancing, I knew I could make a difference in my community, and perhaps even the world.

Epilogue: Today in Guinea, artists are facing huge challenges due to COVID-19. Dancers and musicians typically make the bulk of their money through performing at weddings and other large events, which are now on hold. Sarah Lee is currently hosting a fundraiser called "Rice for Ramadan," and has been delivering foodstuffs to ballets around Conakry. To learn more or donate, visit https://www.gofundme.com/f/rice-for-ramadan.

Recommended resources:

Camp Fareta Guinea. (n.d.). Retrieved July 07, 2020, from https://www.campfaretaguinea.com/

Cohen. (2011). Stages in Transition: Les Ballets Africains and Independence, 1959 to 1960. *Journal of Black Studies, 43*(1), 11-48. doi:10.1177/0021934711426628

Cohen, A. J. (2016). Inalienable Performances, Mutable Heirlooms: Dance, Cultural Inheritance, and Political Transformation in the Republic of Guinea. *American Ethnologist, 43*(4), 650-662. doi:10.1111/amet.12381

Kalani, & Camara, R. M. (2006). *West African Drum & Dance: A Yankadi-Macrou Celebration.* Van Nuys, CA: Alfred.

Price. (2013). Rhythms of culture: Djembe and african memory in african-american cultural traditions. *Black Music Research Journal, 33*(2), 227. doi:10.5406/blacmusiresej.33.2.0227

SUBMIT A STORY
FOR THE NEXT ANTHOLOGY

Submission period: November 1–December 20, 2020

If you're interested in submitting a story, please first read through the section titled "Our Commitments" at the beginning of this book. Works that do not align with these principles will not be considered.

Instructions for submitting a story:

- Stories must be between 1,500 and 3,000 words in length, double spaced, and in 12-point, Times New Roman font
- Stories must fit within one of the following themes: far-out adventure, unexpected opportunities, community, lessons learned, cross-cultural friendships, love stories, or personal development. Please mention the theme of your story in your submission email
- Submissions must include the author's full name, story theme, email address, and phone number at the top
- A title may be included, but is not required
- Multiple submissions from a single author will be reviewed for possible publication, but we ask that rejected stories not be resubmitted except at our express request
- Submissions may be shared via Google Drive with megan@megantaylormorrison.com or sent directly to the same email address. Stories sent via email must be in .doc, .docx, or .rtf format

We will do our best to respond to submissions within 30 days of receipt. If your work is accepted, we will not own its copyright. We do, however, require all our authors to sign a contract ceding us the right to print and distribute their stories.

If we believe your story has promise but needs rewrites, we will recommend that you work with our team of editors to complete it. Please be aware that all submitted works will be subject to editing and proofreading to fit the book's style and content requirements.

Work with our team:

This is a great option if you are new to writing non-fiction short stories. To learn more, send an email to megan@megantaylormorrison.com with the subject line, "Dance Story Consulting." Include your name, your phone number, and a brief description of the story you want to tell. We will contact you within 30 days.

Please note that choosing to collaborate with our editors does not guarantee that your story will be included in the next anthology.

Are you wondering what it's like to work with us?

Check out the following testimonials from 2020 authors about writing in cooperation with Senior Editor Megan Taylor Morrison.

"Over the past few weeks, I've had the extreme pleasure of working with Meg on Dance Adventures. She is a true gem who exudes all the qualities of a leader and visionary. She is patient. She is kind. But most importantly, you can feel her deep love for what she does and her great appreciation for showcasing others. Her selflessness is truly unmatched. Working with her helped me grow in ways I hadn't expected. She allowed me to reminisce and think about my life like I never had before. Meg's attention to detail and curiosity about the intricate moments of life have made her one of the most wonderful people I've had the honor to work with. If you get an opportunity to collaborate with her, do not pass it up. It is life changing."

—*Courtney Celeste Spears, author of "Make Me Proud, Ms. Courts..."*

"I learned so much about storytelling, including how to bring readers into a moment with me. With Meg's help, I've created a story that I love, and that people can connect with."

–Zsuzsi Kapas, author of "Inter-Independence."

"I really enjoyed going through the writing process with Meg. I loved how her edits guided and clarified my voice."

–Laurie Bonner-Baker, author of "The Accidental Audition"

"Working with Meg was a wonderful experience. I was incredibly nervous about participating in this endeavor. Meg was supportive and very encouraging, leading me to feel optimistic about the potential of my story and comfortable speaking with her about what makes me feel vulnerable. Meg made the process easy and fun. I'm so grateful to have had the opportunity to collaborate with her."

–Khalila Fordham, author of "I Am Here"

"Meg's patience, creativity, and passion allowed my writing to become more vibrant and engaging without sacrificing any of my story."

–Alex Milweski, author of "Dancing in the Dunes"

"It was a pleasure to team up with Meg to make sure my story was not only factually precise, but also fun to read. I learned a lot about writing through this process."

–Kara Nepomuceno, author of "A Month in Manila"

"Meg always had awesome suggestions about ways to make my story better, and I liked how she gave specific deadlines and reminded me gently when I needed to finish something."

–Carolyn McPherson, author of "Exploring Kizomba in Angola."

ABOUT THE EDITORS

Meet Senior Editor Megan Taylor Morrison:

In January 2015, a year after returning from Guinea, Megan Taylor Morrison finally took the leap into entrepreneurship. Her first two ventures – a life and business coaching practice, and a travel company called Dance Adventures – have since supported thousands of people in reconnecting to their creativity, confidence, and sense of play, as well as in reaching new levels of personal and professional success.

Meg served as the CEO of Dance Adventures from 2015 to 2018. During her tenure, she created and co-led dance trips to numerous countries, including a collaboration with four-time Emmy® Award-winning television host Mickela Mallozzi on a tango trip to Argentina. In partnership with Melaina Spitzer, she debuted the talk, "Dance Travel: The Next Era of Dance Education," at the National Dance Education Organization's Conference in 2018.

Meg continues to lead trips abroad each year as an independent tour guide, and has served as a dance travel consultant for organizations such as Joy of Motion Dance Center (Washington, DC, USA) and the Maryland Dance Education Association (Towson, MD). The majority of her time, however, is devoted to coaching.

In her private practice, as well as through her speaking engagements and workshops, Meg has supported more than 5,000 clients in achieving their goals, honing their leadership skills, and creating a values-based lifestyle. Meg's work has been featured in *The New York Times*, *The Huffington Post*, *USA Today*, *Yahoo!*, and numerous other publications.

Outside of her work, dancing remains Meg's biggest passion. After studying movement in 15 countries on six continents, she has found that her favorite styles are those created by Black communities in

Harlem during America's jazz era. Meg has had the honor of learning those dances from many teachers, including original lindy hoppers Frankie Manning and Dawn Hampton, and has been an avid performer, competitor, and instructor since 2009. In particular, she has loved teaching about the African roots of solo vernacular jazz at The Process and the NDEO Jazz Conference (Richmond, VA; Newport, RI), competing at the International Lindy Hop Championships (Washington, DC), and dancing with various performance troupes in New York City.

Meg holds a certificate in coaching through Accomplishment Coaching, a Master's in journalism from Northwestern University, and a BA in international affairs and French from the University of Puget Sound.

It's been Meg's great pleasure to serve as the senior editor of this anthology, which was created to honor Dance Adventures' legacy. She hopes that, through the stories in this book, many more people will discover the magic of dance travel.

Meet Assistant Editor Elisa Koshkina:

Since childhood, Elisa Koshkina has been a believer in the vital importance of precise, considerate communication between cultures. After receiving her education in the US and Russia, she worked as an English teacher in Moscow before joining the staff of *Expert Magazine Online* as the senior translator and editor for the English version of the website.

Following the 2008 economic crash, Elisa lived in Latvia and Turkey before returning to the United States. She now works as a freelance provider of translations from Russian, Ukrainian, Spanish, French, and Portuguese to English, as well as English-language editing, proofreading and copywriting services. In 2011, Elisa was awarded the title of Freelancer of the Year by one of her clients, Eclectic Translations.

Elisa primarily specializes in medical and legal translations, viewing these as the best opportunity to provide much-needed assistance to people in difficult situations. She does, however, enjoy working on the occasional creative project. Her collaborations with Munich-based publishing house Manufaktur für Grafikdesign have resulted in two multilingual gift-edition books, *The Painter of Mount Aconcagua* and *The Lands of the Amazons*, the latter of which was a finalist for the Russian Geographical Society's Crystal Compass Award and received first prize in the category of Best Book by a Russian Publisher Abroad from the Russian Publishers Association in 2015.

With three World Figure Championships under her belt, Elisa's primary physical outlet is ice skating. Over the years, her training has been supplemented with lessons in ballet, tap, jazz, contemporary, ballroom, salsa, swing, krump, house, breaking, and popping and locking. Each dance style has made a valuable contribution to both her approach to movement on the ice and her understanding of other artists.

Working on *Dance Adventures* has allowed Elisa to bring several of her passions together in a new, unexpected format, and she has found echoes of her own experiences abroad in many of the anthology's stories. Elisa has derived great joy from helping the authors of *Dance Adventures* relate their unique and highly personal explorations of the intersections between dance, communication, culture, and individual development.

Elisa holds a certificate in Russian language from Lomonosov Moscow State University, a BA in Russian culture from Carleton College, an MA in Buddhist studies/Sanskrit track from Naropa University, and a certificate in teaching English as a foreign language from One World Training. She can be contacted at marketenglish@gmail.com.

"The big question is whether you are going to say a hearty 'yes' to your adventure."
—*Joseph Campbell*

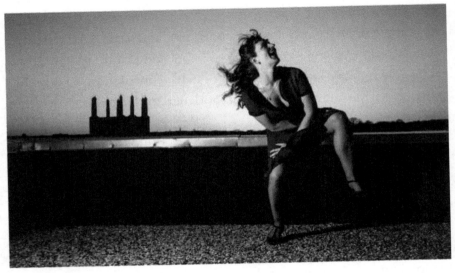

Megan Taylor Morrison, senior editor of Dance Adventures, does solo Charleston on a rooftop in Washington, DC
Photo credit: Jerry Almonte

CPSIA information can be obtained
at www.ICGtesting.com
Printed in the USA
LVHW050336281120
672641LV00005B/253